The Ultimate Guide to
Parasite Cleanse

Natural Methods, Nutritional Plans and Home Remedies
To Treat, Eliminate and Prevent Parasites
For People, Children Pets and Travelers

Liv Marwin

TABLE OF CONTENT

PREFACE 6

1. INTRODUCTION TO PARASITE CLEANSE 7

WHAT IS PARASITOSIS? 8
   Parasitosis: The Hidden Invaders 8
WHY IS PARASITE CLEANSE IMPORTANT? 9

2. INTRODUCTION TO THE HISTORY OF NATURAL PARASITE CLEANSE 10

ANCIENT PARASITE CLEANSE PRACTICES 11
EVOLUTION OF NATURAL METHODS OVER TIME 12
CULTURAL INFLUENCES ON CLEANSE TECHNIQUES 13

3. UNDERSTANDING PARASITES 15

TYPES OF PARASITES 16
   Protozoa 16
   Ectoparasites 18
   Endoparasites 19
   Other Parasites 21
SYMPTOMS AND DIAGNOSIS 22
   Common Symptoms of Parasitic Infections 22
   Tests and Diagnosis: How to Identify Parasites 24

4. PREPARING FOR PARASITE CLEANSE 29

ASSESSING PERSONAL HEALTH 29
   Self-Assessment and Mental Preparation 30
   Consultation with a Healthcare Professional 30
PRE-CLEANSE DIET AND NUTRITION 31
   Foods to Avoid 31
   Foods that Support Parasite Cleanse 32
EVALUATING RISKS AND PRECAUTIONS 35
   Potential Risks of Natural Cleanse Methods 35
   Contraindications for Pre-Existing Health Conditions 36
   When to Consult a Healthcare Professional 37
   Interactions with Medications and Other Treatments 37

5. INTRODUCTION NATURAL PARASITE CLEANSE METHODS 39

HERBS AND SUPPLEMENTS 40
   Aloe Vera 40
   Anise 40
   Barberry 41
   Berberine 41
   Black Walnut Hull 41
   Burdock Root 41
   Castor Oil 42
   Cayenne Pepper 42
   Chamomile 42
   Chlorophyll 42
   Cilantro (Coriander) 42
   Cloves 43
   Coconut Oil 43
   Diatomaceous Earth 43
   Echinacea 43
   Epazote 43
   Fenugreek Seeds 44

Garlic 44
Ginger 44
Goldenseal 44
Grapefruit Seed Extract 44
Holy Basil (Tulsi) 45
Mimosa Pudica 45
Neem 45
Olive Leaf Extract 45
Oregano 45
Papaya Seeds 45
Pau d'Arco 46
Probiotics 46
Pumpkin Seeds 46
Quassia 46
Senna 46
Tansy 46
Thyme 47
Turmeric 47
Wormseed (Chenopodium) 47
Wormwood 47
OTHER NATURAL METHODS 47
Oil Pulling with Coconut Oil 47
Coffee Enemas 48
Bentonite Clay 48
Colloidal Silver Water 49
Water and Salt Cleansing 49

6. PARASITE CLEANSE PROTOCOL 50

RECIPES AND HOME REMEDIES 51
Breakfast Recipes for the Parasite Cleanse 51
Lunch Recipes for the Parasite Cleanse 55
Dinner Recipes for the Parasite Cleanse 60
Snack Recipes for the Parasite Cleanse 66
Teas & Infusions for Parasite Cleanse 71
PARASITE CLEANSE PROGRAM 74
30-Day Program: Step by Step 75
Maintenance Program 83

7. MANAGING SIDE EFFECTS 85

DIE-OFF REACTIONS AND HOW TO MANAGE THEM 85
Understanding Die-Off Reactions 85
Strategies to Mitigate Side Effects 86
IMMUNE SYSTEM SUPPORT 88
Immune-Boosting Supplements 88
Stress Reduction Techniques 90

8. LONG-TERM PARASITE CLEANSE AND PREVENTION 93

MAINTAINING A PARASITE-FREE BODY 94
Healthy Eating Habits 94
Regular Cleansing Routines 95
HYGIENE AND LIFESTYLE 96
Tips for a Clean Home Environment 96
Preventing Reinfections 97
ADVANCED NATURAL PREVENTION 98
Strengthening the Immune System Naturally 98
Long-Term Anti-Parasitic Diet 99
Preventive Use of Herbs and Supplements 99
Periodic Detoxification Techniques 100

ADVICE FOR TRAVELERS 100
  Natural Preparation Before Travel.. 100
  Herbs and Supplements to Carry While Traveling.. 101
  Hygiene Practices During Travel... 102
  Managing Diet in High-Risk Countries.. 102
  Post-Travel Natural Cleansing... 103

9. PARASITE CLEANSE FOR CHILDREN AND PETS 104

PARASITE CLEANSE FOR CHILDREN 105
  Specific Symptoms in Children.. 105
  Safe and Natural Methods for Kids... 105
  Diet and Nutrition for Children... 106
  Example Meal Plan for Children... 107
PARASITE CLEANSE FOR PETS 108
  Symptoms and Diagnosis in Dogs and Cats.. 108
  Natural Cleansing Methods for Pets.. 109
  Prevention and Maintenance of Pet Health... 110

10. UNDERSTANDING AND MANAGING EXTERNAL PARASITES 112

TYPES OF EXTERNAL PARASITES.. 112
SYMPTOMS AND IDENTIFICATION 113
  Signs of External Parasitic Infections.. 114
  Diagnostic Techniques... 114
NATURAL TREATMENTS FOR EXTERNAL PARASITES 115
  Herbal Sprays and Washes.. 115
  Essential Oils for Topical Use... 116
  Natural Preventative Measures... 116
LONG-TERM PREVENTION... 117
  Maintaining a Clean Living Environment.. 117
  Regular Inspection and Early Detection.. 118
  Natural Preventative Measures... 118

11. PSYCHO-EMOTIONAL SUPPORT DURING PARASITE CLEANSE 120

MANAGING STRESS AND ANXIETY.. 120
MINDFULNESS AND MEDITATION TECHNIQUES 120
EMOTIONAL SUPPORT DURING THE CLEANSING PROCESS............................. 121
INCORPORATING SELF-CARE PRACTICES 121

12. CONCLUSION 122

REFLECTIONS ON THE IMPORTANCE OF NATURAL PARASITE CLEANSE............. 122
CALL TO ACTION AND CONTINUED AWARENESS.. 123

ACKNOWLEDGMENTS 124

APPENDIX 125

GLOSSARY OF TERMS.. 125
ANTI-PARASITIC NUTRITIONAL GUIDE.. 126

Preface

In our modern world, health often takes a backseat to our busy lives. Yet, one often overlooked aspect of well-being is the impact of parasites on our bodies. These tiny invaders can affect our health in subtle ways, leading to a range of symptoms that are frequently misunderstood or ignored.

This book explores natural methods to cleanse and protect our bodies from parasites. It combines traditional wisdom with current scientific understanding to provide a comprehensive guide to parasite cleansing and prevention. The information within these pages aims to empower you to take charge of your health using time-tested natural approaches.

We'll journey through various aspects of parasite cleansing, starting with understanding what parasites are and how they affect us. We'll explore the history of natural cleansing practices and delve into safe, effective methods suitable for everyone, including children and pets.

You'll find detailed protocols for thorough parasite cleansing, including recipes and home remedies. We'll also discuss supporting your body during the cleanse, managing side effects, and maintaining long-term health. The book covers both internal and external parasites, offering practical advice for a clean, parasite-free environment.

For travelers, we provide guidelines to help you stay healthy on your journeys. We also touch on the importance of emotional and mental support during a cleanse, encouraging a holistic approach to healing.

This book is an invitation to a healthier, more vibrant life. By integrating these natural methods into your routine, you're making a commitment to your well-being. May this serve as your companion on the path to better health.

1. Introduction to Parasite Cleanse

Parasites might be one of the most underestimated threats to our health today. While many assume these unwelcome invaders are a problem only in distant, less developed regions, the truth is that parasites affect billions of people worldwide, across all continents. In fact, it's estimated that around **3.5 billion people** are infected with at least one type of parasitic organism. Whether it's a child playing in the backyard, a pet sleeping on the couch, or a traveler exploring new places, no one is entirely safe from these hidden dangers.

The Ultimate Guide to Parasite Cleanse is here to open your eyes to the realities of parasitic infections and provide you with the knowledge and tools you need to protect yourself and your loved ones. This book delves into the fascinating world of parasites, exploring how they operate and the often subtle symptoms they cause. You will learn about natural methods, nutritional plans, and effective home remedies to treat, eliminate, and prevent parasites from taking hold.

Imagine regaining control of your health, boosting your energy, and living free from the discomfort and anxiety that parasites can bring. By understanding the nature of these unseen invaders and adopting proactive cleansing routines, you can enhance your well-being and ensure a healthier future. Dive into this guide and embark on a journey towards a parasite-free life—your body will thank you.

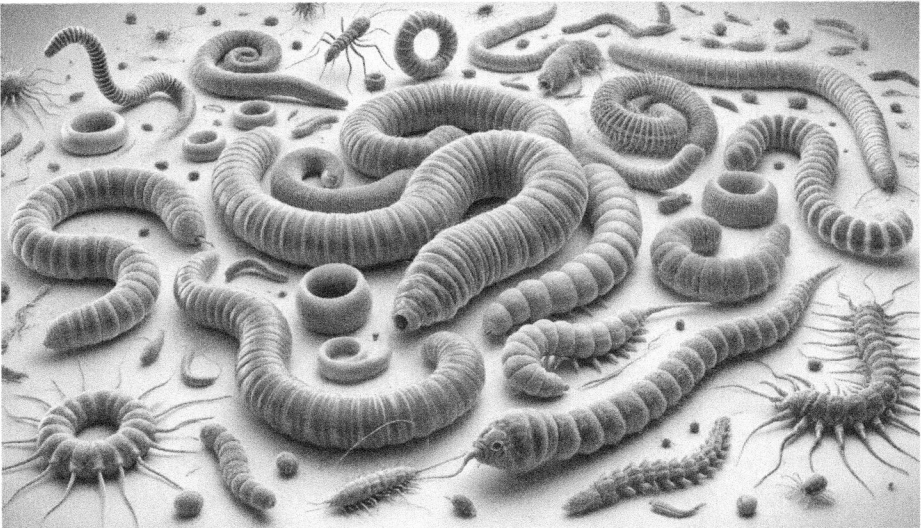

WHAT IS PARASITOSIS?

Parasitosis, derived from the Greek "para" (beside) and "sitos" (food), is a medical condition characterized by the infestation of a host organism by parasites. Scientifically, it refers to a symbiotic relationship in which one organism (the parasite) lives on or within another organism (the host), obtaining nutrients and shelter at the host's expense, often resulting in harm or disease to the host.

Parasitosis: The Hidden Invaders

Parasitosis isn't just a problem in far-off lands; it's a health issue that hits closer to home than most realize. At its core, parasitosis is an infestation of organisms that live off their hosts, sapping nutrients and causing a range of health problems.

These freeloaders come in three main flavors: protozoa, helminths, and ectoparasites. Protozoa are single-celled troublemakers that can multiply inside you, causing diseases like malaria or giardiasis. Helminths, or worms, are the multi-celled squatters that set up shop in your gut and beyond. Think tapeworms and roundworms - some can grow as long as your forearm. Ectoparasites like ticks and lice are the external hitchhikers, hitching a ride on your skin and potentially transmitting nasty diseases.

The kicker? Parasitosis often flies under the radar. Its symptoms - gut issues, constant fatigue, weird rashes, unexplained weight loss - mimic other conditions, making diagnosis a real head-scratcher. And forget the notion that parasites only plague developing countries. These equal-opportunity invaders can affect anyone, anywhere.

Parasites are master evaders, often outmaneuvering the body's defenses. They've honed their survival skills over millennia, allowing them to thrive where they're not welcome. The impact on health can be subtle at first but potentially devastating over time.

Here's the real eye-opener: parasites don't discriminate. Your posh neighborhood or fancy bottled water won't necessarily protect you. Travel, pets, contaminated food - even a simple handshake - can be all it takes for these microscopic menaces to find a new home.

Understanding parasitosis is crucial in our interconnected world. By recognizing the signs and ditching the stigma, we can tackle these infections head-on. In the battle against these tiny terrors, knowledge isn't just power - it's your best defense.

WHY IS PARASITE CLEANSE IMPORTANT?

Parasite cleansing isn't just another health fad—it's a vital reset for your body's ecosystem. These microscopic squatters can wreak havoc on your health, often in ways you might not immediately connect to parasitic infection. From chronic fatigue to unexplained weight loss, these invaders can quietly undermine your well-being.

In our modern world, we're more vulnerable to parasites than we'd like to admit. Processed foods, high-stress lifestyles, and limited connection with nature create a perfect storm for these opportunistic organisms. Even mundane activities like petting your dog or eating out can be gateways for parasitic invasion.

A proper cleanse isn't about quick fixes; it's about reclaiming control of your internal environment. By targeting these freeloaders, you're not just addressing symptoms—you're tackling root causes. This proactive approach can lead to improved digestion, enhanced nutrient absorption, and a significant boost in energy levels.

Moreover, eliminating parasites takes a load off your immune system. When your body isn't constantly battling these invaders, it can redirect its resources to overall health maintenance and disease prevention. The result? Clearer thinking, better sleep, and a renewed sense of vitality.

Regular cleansing is like performing routine maintenance on a car—it keeps your body running smoothly and prevents long-term damage. It's an investment in your future health, potentially warding off chronic conditions linked to prolonged parasitic infections.

There's also a psychological benefit to cleansing. Knowing you've taken active steps to purge these unwanted guests can bring a sense of empowerment and mental clarity. In our high-stress world, this peace of mind is invaluable.

Embracing natural cleansing methods aligns with a holistic approach to health. Unlike harsh pharmaceuticals, natural remedies support your body's innate cleansing mechanisms without the risk of harmful side effects.

In essence, parasite cleansing is about optimization—creating an internal environment where your body can thrive. It's not just about eliminating parasites; it's about cultivating vibrant health from the inside out.

2. Introduction to the History of Natural Parasite Cleanse

Natural parasite cleansing has been a crucial part of human history across various cultures. Confronted with parasitic infections, our ancestors relied on the natural world, utilizing plants, herbs, and other substances long before modern medicine. These remedies were deeply rooted in the spiritual, cultural, and environmental contexts of their times.

In ancient civilizations, knowledge of parasite cleansing was carefully documented and passed down. Traditional Chinese Medicine, for example, contains numerous herbal remedies designed to expel parasites and promote health, while Ayurveda in India emphasizes natural ingredients like neem and turmeric. Native American practices also demonstrate a deep understanding of local flora, using plants with anti-parasitic properties alongside spiritual rituals that connect body, mind, and spirit.

Throughout history, these ancient methods have influenced modern approaches to natural health, illustrating human ingenuity and a continuous search for sustainable health solutions. The renewed interest in these traditional practices today highlights their lasting relevance and potential for addressing contemporary health challenges, providing insights into the holistic perspectives that have shaped our understanding of wellness.

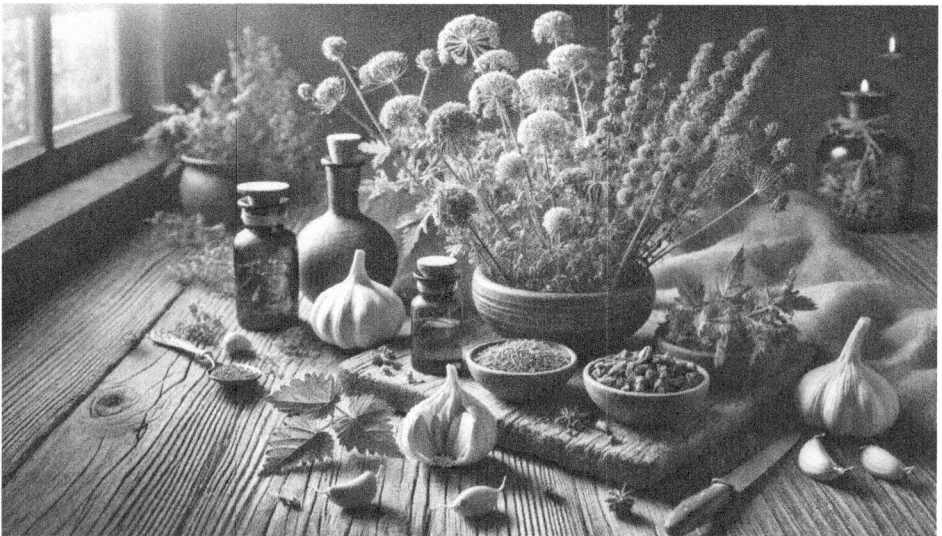

ANCIENT PARASITE CLEANSE PRACTICES

Parasite cleansing is deeply rooted in ancient medical traditions across various cultures, offering a wealth of natural remedies that remain relevant today. These time-honored practices reflect centuries of knowledge in combating parasitic infections and emphasize the holistic nature of health.

In Traditional Chinese Medicine (TCM), the approach to parasite cleansing is holistic, focusing on restoring balance within the body. TCM practitioners believe that parasites thrive in environments where internal imbalances, such as dampness and heat, are present. Treatments are designed not only to expel parasites but also to correct these underlying conditions. Key herbs in TCM include Wormwood, known for its potent anti-parasitic properties, Garlic, Pumpkin Seeds, and Coptis. These herbs are often combined in specific formulations to maximize their effectiveness. Additionally, acupuncture and dietary therapy play supportive roles in TCM, stimulating the immune system and promoting a diet that creates an inhospitable environment for parasites.

Indian Ayurveda, one of the oldest holistic health systems, also places great emphasis on parasite cleansing. Ayurveda views health as a balance of the three doshas: Vata, Pitta, and Kapha. Parasitic infections are often attributed to an excess of Kapha, which provides a favorable environment for parasites. Ayurvedic treatments include powerful herbs like Neem, Vidanga, and Triphala, known for their anti-parasitic properties. Panchakarma, the Ayurvedic detoxification process, includes procedures such as therapeutic vomiting, purgation, enemas, and bloodletting, all tailored to the individual's constitution. This comprehensive approach not only eliminates parasites but also restores overall balance.

In Native American traditions, parasite cleansing is closely tied to spiritual and natural elements. Health is seen as a state of harmony with nature, and illness as a disruption of this balance. Native healers use plants like Black Walnut, Wormwood, and Goldenseal for their anti-parasitic effects. These remedies are often combined with spiritual practices such as smudging with sage and cedar, which are believed to purify the body and spirit. These rituals highlight the belief that true healing involves restoring harmony at both the physical and spiritual levels.

Ancient practices emphasize nature's healing power and maintaining bodily balance for parasite cleansing. By integrating natural remedies with a holistic understanding of the body, these traditions offer valuable insights for improving modern approaches to managing parasitic infections.

EVOLUTION OF NATURAL METHODS OVER TIME

The evolution of natural parasite cleanse methods showcases humanity's ingenuity and resilience in addressing health challenges. From ancient herbal remedies to modern holistic practices, this journey reflects an ongoing quest to harness nature's power for well-being.

In the early days, treatments were largely empirical, based on observation and trial and error. Ancient healers identified plants and substances with anti-parasitic properties through keen observation. These foundational practices laid the groundwork for more systematic approaches that would develop over time.

The advent of modern science in the 19th and 20th centuries brought a significant shift. The discovery of microorganisms and germ theory revolutionized medicine, leading to the development of pharmaceutical anti-parasitic drugs. However, natural remedies remained widely used, especially where access to modern medicine was limited.

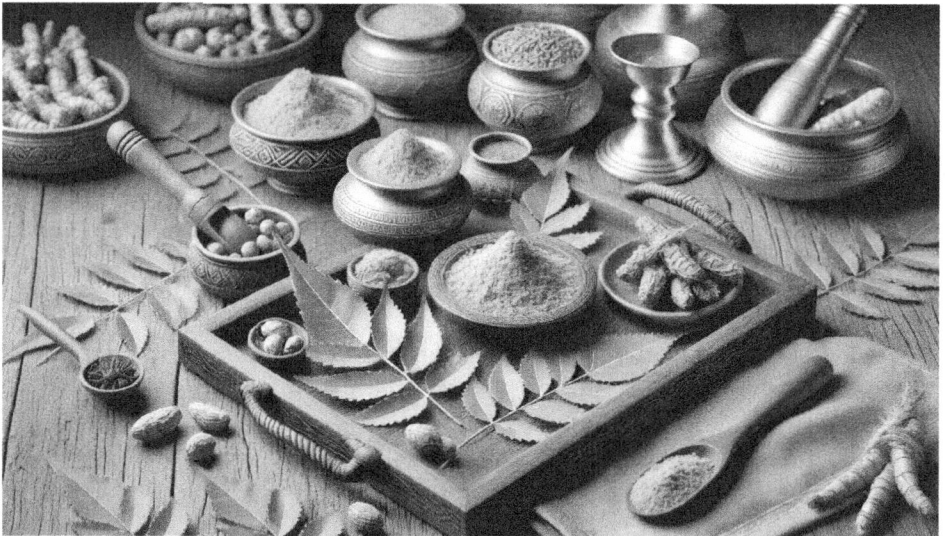

During the late 20th century, a holistic health movement emerged, integrating traditional knowledge with scientific understanding. Herbalists and naturopaths began systematically documenting and validating the efficacy of traditional remedies, bridging the gap between ancient wisdom and modern science.

The integration of holistic practices into mainstream health care has also played a crucial role. Personalized approaches, such as detoxification protocols and dietary modifications, are now commonly recommended, supporting the body's natural healing processes.

Moreover, the rise of global health awareness and the focus on preventive care have emphasized the importance of maintaining a parasite-free body. Regular cleansing, healthy diets, and good hygiene are recognized as essential components of overall wellness.

The evolution of natural parasite cleanse methods represents a convergence of ancient wisdom, modern science, and holistic health practices. This dynamic process reflects a broader trend towards integrative health care, where traditional remedies are validated through research and modern practices are enriched by historical knowledge. As we continue to explore and refine these methods, we become better equipped to address the challenges of parasitic infections in a holistic and sustainable manner.

CULTURAL INFLUENCES ON CLEANSE TECHNIQUES

Cultural influences have profoundly shaped the development and adoption of parasite cleanse techniques throughout history. Different cultures, with their unique beliefs, traditions, and environmental contexts, have contributed to a diverse array of methods for combating parasitic infections. These practices highlight human ingenuity and the importance of integrating traditional knowledge with modern healthcare.

In indigenous cultures, natural remedies for parasite cleansing are deeply rooted in their connection to the environment. Native American tribes, for example, have long used regional plants and herbs for medicinal purposes. The Cherokee used black walnut hulls, while the Lakota relied on sagebrush for cleansing. These practices were intertwined with spiritual beliefs and respect for nature.

Traditional Chinese Medicine (TCM) also has a rich history of using herbal remedies to address parasitic infections. TCM views health holistically, considering the balance of energies within the body. Herbs such as wormwood and ginger are staples in TCM for their ability to expel parasites and restore balance. TCM encompasses diet, lifestyle, and preventive measures, reflecting a comprehensive approach to health.

In India, Ayurveda emphasizes maintaining balance through diet, lifestyle, and herbal treatments. Ancient texts detail remedies for parasitic infections, including neem, turmeric, and triphala. Ayurveda categorizes individuals into doshas and tailors treatments accordingly, reflecting a nuanced understanding of health in Indian culture.

African traditional medicine also showcases extensive knowledge of parasite cleansing. Healers in various African communities use plants like Artemisia and papaya seeds for their anti-parasitic properties. Traditional medicine in Africa is often communal, with healers playing a crucial role in community health. The integration of traditional and modern medicine highlights the relevance and effectiveness of these practices.

In South America, indigenous groups rely on the Amazon rainforest's biodiversity for medicinal needs. Plants like epazote and pau d'arco have been used for centuries to treat parasitic infections. This knowledge is intertwined with cultural practices and spiritual beliefs, viewing health as harmony between the individual, community, and environment.

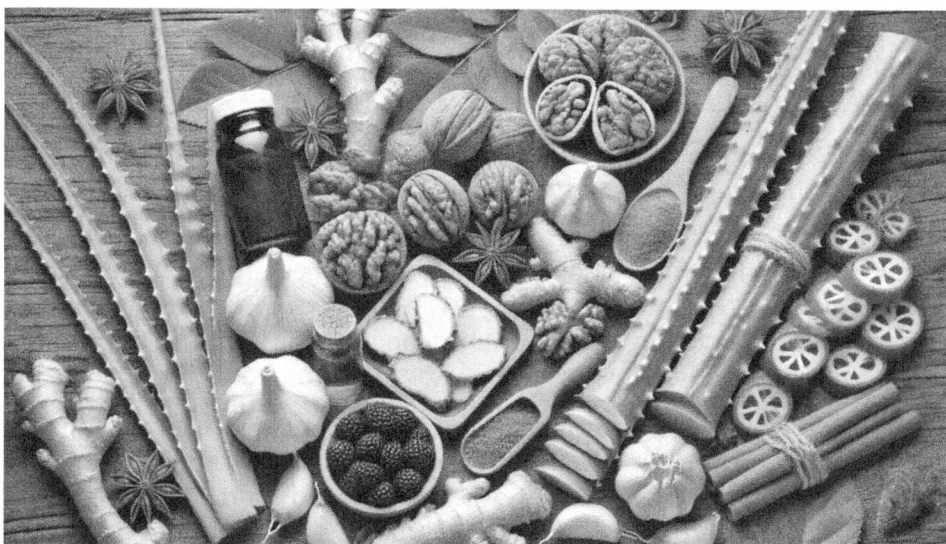

Western culture has also influenced parasite cleanse techniques, particularly through the holistic health movement in the 20th century. This movement embraced natural remedies and traditional practices, integrating them into mainstream healthcare. The growing recognition of their value reflects a desire for natural and sustainable health practices.

Cultural influences on parasite cleanse techniques underscore the rich tapestry of human knowledge. They highlight the importance of preserving traditional practices while integrating them into modern healthcare. Exploring and validating these methods provides a deeper understanding of the interconnectedness of health, culture, and the environment. The diverse approaches remind us that effective treatments often come from blending traditional wisdom with contemporary science.

3. Understanding Parasites

Parasites are silent invaders, often undetected until they've caused significant harm to their hosts. This chapter explores the complex world of parasites, providing insights into their types, life cycles, and the health issues they can cause.

Parasites fall into three main categories: protozoa (microscopic single-celled organisms), ectoparasites (living on the host's surface), and endoparasites (inhabiting internal organs and tissues). Each type presents unique challenges, from protozoa causing diseases like malaria to ectoparasites transmitting infections and endoparasites leading to severe internal complications.

The life cycles of these parasites are often intricate, involving multiple hosts and developmental stages, which makes eradication difficult. For example, the malaria parasite requires both humans and mosquitoes to complete its cycle.

Symptoms of parasitic infections are diverse and can mimic other diseases, complicating diagnosis. They range from gastrointestinal issues to neurological symptoms. Accurate identification often requires a combination of clinical evaluation and specific tests.

Natural Diagnostic Methods may include stool analysis, blood tests for antibodies, and muscle testing. These methods can provide initial indications of parasitic presence.

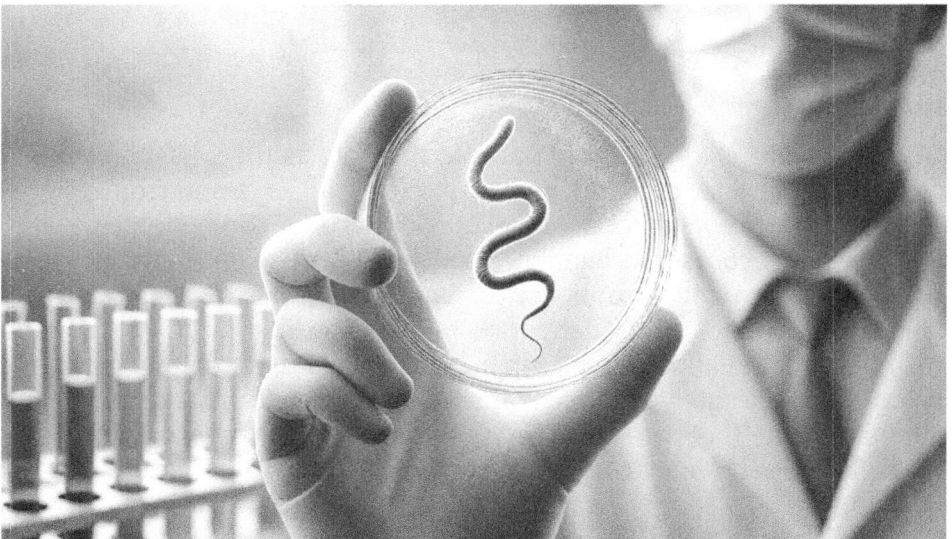

Conventional Diagnostic Methods typically involve laboratory tests such as microscopic examination of stool samples, blood tests, and imaging techniques like MRI or CT scans for more complex cases.

Understanding these aspects of parasites - their types, life cycles, symptoms, and diagnostic methods - is crucial for effective prevention, timely diagnosis, and successful treatment of parasitic infections.

TYPES OF PARASITES

Parasites are organisms that live on or inside another organism, the host, causing harm and deriving sustenance at the host's expense. They come in various forms and sizes, impacting millions of people worldwide. Understanding the different types of parasites is crucial for effective treatment and prevention.

Protozoa

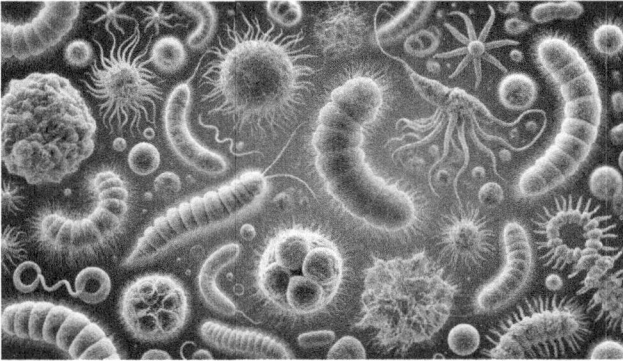

Protozoa are microscopic, single-celled organisms that can reproduce within the human body, leading to various diseases. Here, we will explore some notable protozoa that cause significant health issues.

Giardia

Giardia lamblia is a protozoan parasite that infects the small intestine. It has a simple life cycle involving a cyst and a trophozoite stage. Transmission occurs through ingestion of cysts in contaminated water, food, or direct contact with infected individuals. Once inside the host, the cysts transform into trophozoites, causing symptoms like diarrhea, abdominal cramps, and dehydration. Long-term effects can include malnutrition and impaired growth in children. Natural treatments involve using herbs like garlic, goldenseal, and probiotics to restore gut health and eliminate the parasite. Prevention focuses on consuming clean, filtered water and practicing good hygiene.

Entamoeba histolytica (Amoeba)

Entamoeba histolytica causes amoebiasis, primarily infecting the large intestine. Its life cycle includes cyst and trophozoite stages, similar to Giardia. Infection occurs through ingesting cysts via contaminated food or water. Trophozoites invade the intestinal lining, causing symptoms like dysentery, abdominal pain, and fever. Long-term consequences can include liver abscesses and colitis. Natural remedies for amoebiasis include using turmeric, garlic, and probiotics. Preventive measures involve ensuring food and water safety and maintaining proper sanitation.

Plasmodium (Cause of Malaria)

Plasmodium is the protozoan responsible for malaria, a disease transmitted by the Anopheles mosquito. There are several species of Plasmodium, with P. falciparum being the most deadly. The parasite undergoes a complex life cycle involving the mosquito vector and human host. In humans, it infects liver cells and red blood cells, causing symptoms such as fever, chills, and anemia. Malaria can lead to severe complications, including cerebral malaria and organ failure. Natural treatments for malaria include using artemisinin from the sweet wormwood plant and quinine from the cinchona tree. Prevention involves using mosquito nets, repellents, and antimalarial prophylactics.

Trypanosoma (Cause of Sleeping Sickness)

Trypanosoma brucei causes African trypanosomiasis, also known as sleeping sickness, transmitted by the tsetse fly. The parasite undergoes a complex life cycle between the tsetse fly and the human host. It invades the blood and lymphatic system, causing symptoms like fever, headache, and joint pain. In its advanced stage, it crosses the blood-brain barrier, leading to neurological symptoms and disruption of the sleep cycle. Long-term consequences can include severe neurological damage and death if untreated. Natural treatments focus on using herbs like neem, soursop, and immune-boosting supplements. Preventive measures include wearing protective clothing, using insect repellents, and controlling tsetse fly populations.

Leishmania

Leishmania species cause leishmaniasis, transmitted by the bite of infected sandflies. The parasite has a life cycle involving promastigotes in sandflies and amastigotes in humans. Leishmaniasis manifests in different forms: cutaneous, mucocutaneous, and visceral. Symptoms vary based on the form, ranging from skin ulcers to severe organ damage. Long-term consequences include disfigurement and systemic infection. Natural treatments for leishmaniasis include using tea tree oil, neem, and immune-supporting herbs. Prevention involves avoiding sandfly bites through protective clothing, insect repellents, and environmental management.

Ectoparasites

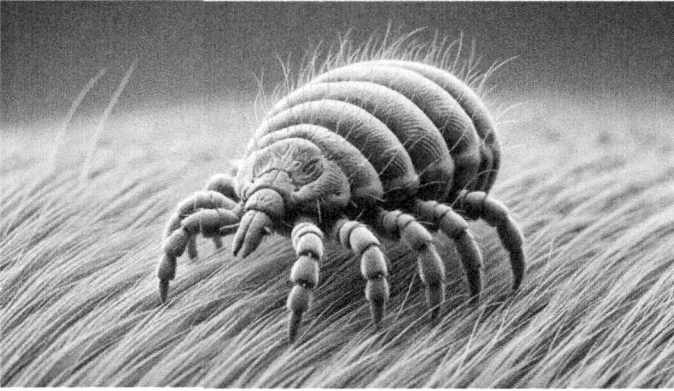

Ectoparasites live on the surface of the host and include organisms like fleas, ticks, lice, and mites. They often cause skin irritation and can transmit other diseases.

Fleas

Fleas are small, wingless insects that feed on the blood of mammals and birds. They have a life cycle consisting of egg, larva, pupa, and adult stages. Fleas can transmit diseases like the bubonic plague and typhus. Symptoms of flea bites include itching, redness, and swelling. Long-term infestations can lead to secondary skin infections. Natural treatments for flea infestations involve using diatomaceous earth, neem oil, and essential oils like lavender and eucalyptus. Prevention includes regular grooming of pets, vacuuming, and using flea repellents.

Ticks

Ticks are arachnids that feed on the blood of mammals, birds, and reptiles. They have a life cycle with egg, larva, nymph, and adult stages. Ticks can transmit diseases like Lyme disease, Rocky Mountain spotted fever, and babesiosis. Symptoms of tick bites include a red spot or rash, itching, and flu-like symptoms. Long-term effects can include chronic joint inflammation and neurological issues. Natural treatments for tick bites include using tea tree oil, apple cider vinegar, and herbal tinctures. Prevention involves wearing protective clothing, using tick repellents, and checking for ticks after outdoor activities.

Lice

Lice are small, wingless insects that live on the scalp and body, feeding on human blood. They have a life cycle with egg (nit), nymph, and adult stages. Lice infestations cause itching, sores, and a crawling sensation on the skin. Long-term infestations can lead to secondary bacterial infections. Natural treatments for lice include using neem oil, tea tree oil, and combing with a fine-toothed comb. Prevention involves maintaining good personal hygiene and avoiding close contact with infested individuals.

Mites (Scabies)

Mites causing scabies burrow into the skin, causing intense itching and rash. They have a life cycle with egg, larva, nymph, and adult stages. Scabies is transmitted through close personal contact or sharing infested items. Symptoms include severe itching, especially at night, and pimple-like rashes. Long-term infestations can lead to skin crusting and secondary infections. Natural treatments for scabies involve using neem oil, tea tree oil, and sulfur ointments. Prevention includes maintaining personal hygiene and avoiding contact with infested individuals.

Endoparasites

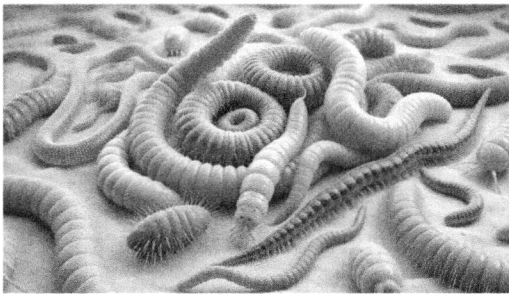

Endoparasites live inside the host, often in the intestines, and include various worms and other organisms.

Intestinal Worms

Intestinal worms are a common type of endoparasite affecting millions worldwide. They can cause malnutrition, abdominal pain, and digestive issues. Examples include ascarids, pinworms, and whipworms.

Ascarids

Ascaris lumbricoides is a large roundworm infecting the human intestine. Its life cycle involves egg, larva, and adult stages. Transmission occurs through ingesting eggs in contaminated food or soil. Symptoms include abdominal pain, malnutrition, and intestinal blockage. Long-term infections can lead to impaired growth in children. Natural treatments involve using papaya seeds, garlic, and wormwood. Prevention includes practicing good hygiene and avoiding contaminated food and water.

Pinworms

Pinworms are small, white worms that infect the intestines, causing intense itching around the anus. They have a life cycle with egg, larva, and adult stages. Transmission occurs through ingesting or inhaling eggs from contaminated surfaces. Symptoms include itching, restlessness, and irritability. Long-term infestations can lead to secondary bacterial infections. Natural treatments involve using garlic, coconut oil, and pumpkin seeds. Prevention includes maintaining good personal hygiene and washing bedding and clothing regularly.

Whipworms

Whipworms are intestinal parasites with a life cycle involving egg, larva, and adult stages. Transmission occurs through ingesting eggs from contaminated soil or food. Symptoms include abdominal pain, diarrhea, and weight loss. Long-term infections can lead to anemia and growth retardation in children. Natural treatments involve using neem, turmeric, and probiotics. Prevention includes practicing good hygiene and ensuring food safety.

Anisakis

Anisakis is a parasitic worm found in marine fish and squid. Its life cycle involves egg, larva, and adult stages. Transmission occurs through consuming raw or undercooked seafood. Symptoms include abdominal pain, nausea, and vomiting. Long-term infections can cause gastrointestinal issues. Natural treatments involve using garlic, ginger, and probiotics. Prevention includes avoiding raw or undercooked seafood and freezing fish before consumption.

Flatworms

Flatworms include tapeworms and flukes, which can infect the intestines and other organs. They have complex life cycles involving intermediate hosts like snails or fish.

Tapeworms (Taenia)

Tapeworms are long, flat worms that live in the intestines. They have a life cycle involving egg, larva, and adult stages. Transmission occurs through ingesting eggs or larvae in contaminated food, especially undercooked meat. Symptoms include abdominal pain, weight loss, and malnutrition. Long-term infections can lead to nutrient deficiencies and digestive issues. Natural treatments involve using garlic, pumpkin seeds, and papaya seeds. Prevention includes cooking meat thoroughly and practicing good food hygiene.

Schistosoma

Schistosoma is a parasitic flatworm causing schistosomiasis. Its life cycle involves freshwater snails as intermediate hosts. Transmission occurs through contact with contaminated water. Symptoms include rash, fever, and abdominal pain. Long-term infections can lead to liver and kidney damage. Natural treatments involve using turmeric, garlic, and immune-boosting herbs. Prevention includes avoiding contact with contaminated water and using protective clothing.

Roundworms

Roundworms are cylindrical worms that infect the intestines and other organs. They include species like Ascaris lumbricoides and Toxocara canis.

Ascaris lumbricoides

Ascaris lumbricoides is a large roundworm infecting the intestines. Its life cycle involves egg, larva, and adult stages. Transmission occurs through ingesting eggs in contaminated food or soil. Symptoms include abdominal pain, malnutrition, and intestinal blockage. Long-term infections can lead to impaired growth in children. Natural treatments involve using papaya seeds, garlic, and wormwood. Prevention includes practicing good hygiene and avoiding contaminated food and water.

Toxocara canis

Toxocara canis is a roundworm infecting dogs and humans. Its life cycle involves egg, larva, and adult stages. Transmission occurs through ingesting eggs from contaminated soil or dog feces. Symptoms include fever, coughing, and abdominal pain. Long-term infections can lead to organ damage and vision loss. Natural treatments involve using neem, turmeric, and immune-supporting herbs. Prevention includes deworming pets and practicing good hygiene.

Other Parasites

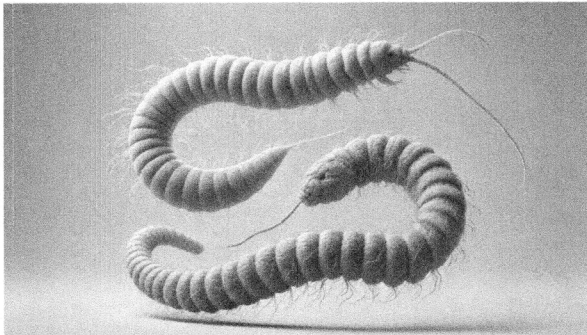

Strongyloides stercoralis

Strongyloides stercoralis is a parasitic roundworm infecting the intestines. Its life cycle involves egg, larva, and adult stages. Transmission occurs through skin contact with contaminated soil. Symptoms include abdominal pain, diarrhea, and skin rash. Long-term infections can lead to severe malabsorption and immunocompromised states. Natural treatments involve using garlic, turmeric, and immune-boosting supplements. Prevention includes wearing protective footwear and practicing good hygiene.

Trichinella spiralis

Trichinella spiralis is a parasitic roundworm causing trichinosis. Its life cycle involves egg, larva, and adult stages. Transmission occurs through consuming undercooked meat, especially pork. Symptoms include abdominal pain, muscle pain, and fever. Long-term infections can lead to muscle damage and inflammation. Natural treatments involve using garlic, ginger, and immune-supporting herbs. Prevention includes cooking meat thoroughly and practicing good food hygiene.

SYMPTOMS AND DIAGNOSIS

Understanding the symptoms and diagnostic methods for parasitic infections is crucial for timely and effective intervention. Parasites can manifest a wide range of symptoms, depending on the type and location of the infestation. Recognizing these symptoms early can lead to better outcomes and prevent long-term complications.

Common Symptoms of Parasitic Infections

Parasitic infections can present with a variety of symptoms that are often non-specific, making diagnosis challenging. However, certain patterns can help in identifying the presence of parasites in the body.

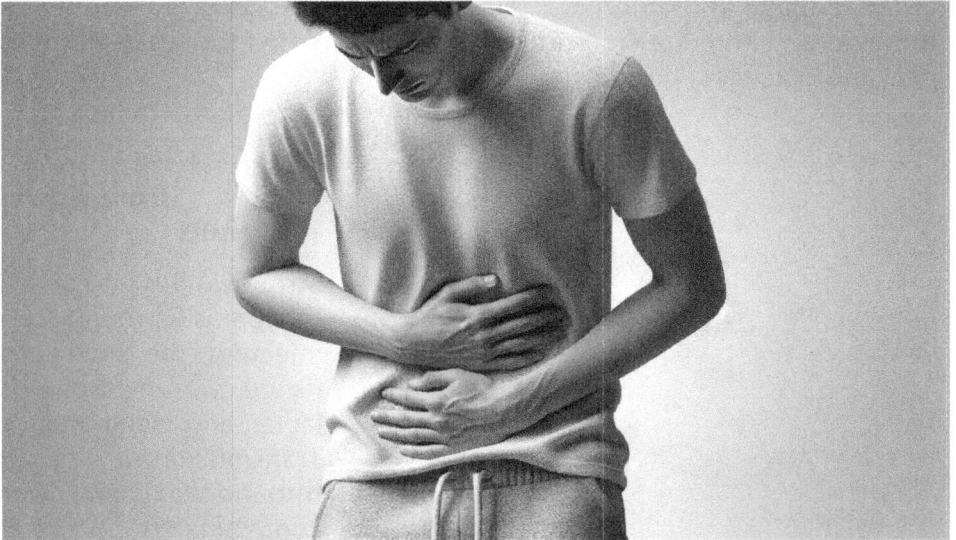

Gastrointestinal Distress

One of the most common signs of parasitic infection is gastrointestinal distress. This includes symptoms such as diarrhea, constipation, gas, bloating, and abdominal pain. These symptoms occur because many parasites reside in the intestines, disrupting normal digestive functions.

For example, Giardia lamblia causes significant abdominal cramps and diarrhea, leading to dehydration and malnutrition.

Unexplained Fatigue

Persistent, unexplained fatigue is another hallmark of parasitic infections. This fatigue results from the body's continuous battle against the parasites, which drain the host's energy and nutrients. For instance, infections caused by Plasmodium (malaria) often lead to severe fatigue due to the destruction of red blood cells, causing anemia.

Skin Issues

Various skin issues can signal a parasitic infection. These include rashes, hives, eczema, and itching. Scabies, caused by mites, is notorious for creating intense itching and a rash that worsens at night. Similarly, hookworm larvae can cause a distinctive rash known as "ground itch" at the site of skin penetration.

Weight Loss and Nutritional Deficiencies

Unexplained weight loss and nutritional deficiencies can also be symptoms of a parasitic infection. Parasites consume the host's nutrients, leading to malnutrition despite an adequate diet. Tapeworms, for example, absorb significant amounts of the host's nutrients, causing weight loss and deficiencies in vitamins and minerals.

Neurological Symptoms

Some parasitic infections can affect the nervous system, leading to neurological symptoms. These can include headaches, seizures, and cognitive disturbances. Neurocysticercosis, caused by the pork tapeworm Taenia solium, can lead to seizures and other severe neurological issues when larvae infect the brain.

Muscle and Joint Pain

Muscle and joint pain can also be indicative of parasitic infections. Trichinella spiralis, responsible for trichinosis, resides in muscle tissue and causes significant muscle pain and inflammation. Similarly, Lyme disease, transmitted by ticks, often presents with joint pain and swelling.

Respiratory Issues

Certain parasites can affect the respiratory system, leading to symptoms like coughing, wheezing, and shortness of breath. Ascaris lumbricoides larvae migrate through the lungs, causing respiratory symptoms during their life cycle. Similarly, Strongyloides stercoralis can cause respiratory distress when larvae migrate through the lungs.

Mental Health Changes

Parasites can also impact mental health, leading to symptoms such as anxiety, depression, and mood swings. The presence of parasites triggers an immune response that can influence neurotransmitter levels, affecting mood and mental well-being. For example, Toxoplasma gondii, associated with toxoplasmosis, has been linked to changes in behavior and increased risk of psychiatric disorders.

Tests and Diagnosis: How to Identify Parasites

Accurate diagnosis of parasitic infections is essential for effective treatment. Both natural and conventional diagnostic methods can help identify the presence of parasites in the body. Understanding the options available can guide you in choosing the best approach for your needs.

NATURAL DIAGNOSTIC METHODS

While not scientifically validated, some natural methods and home remedies are used by individuals as preliminary checks for parasitic infections. These should not replace professional medical diagnostics but can be a starting point for those exploring their health.

Garlic Test

What It Is: Some people believe that consuming raw garlic can help identify a parasitic infection. Garlic is known for its antiparasitic properties, and the theory is that if you experience a die-off reaction (a worsening of symptoms such as bloating, nausea, or fatigue) after consuming raw garlic, it might indicate the presence of parasites.

How It's Done: Eat a small amount of raw garlic and monitor your body's reaction over the next 24-48 hours. Symptoms like increased gas, bloating, or changes in bowel movements are often interpreted by proponents of this method as signs of a parasitic die-off.

Note: This is a highly anecdotal method and not scientifically proven. Reactions to garlic can also be due to other factors, including its strong digestive effects.

Saliva Test

What It Is: This involves checking saliva for cloudiness, which some believe indicates the presence of toxins released by parasites.

How It's Done: Upon waking, before eating or drinking anything, spit into a clear glass of water and let it sit for 15-30 minutes. If the saliva appears stringy or cloudy and sinks to the bottom, it is thought by some to indicate the presence of parasites or an imbalance in gut flora.

Note: There is no scientific basis for this test; it is purely speculative and can be influenced by many factors, including dehydration and the normal breakdown of proteins in saliva.

Tape Test for Pinworms

What It Is: A simple test often recommended for children who are suspected of having pinworms (Enterobius vermicularis), a type of intestinal parasite.

How It's Done: Apply a piece of clear adhesive tape to the skin around the anus in the morning before bathing or using the bathroom. Pinworms often lay eggs at night, and these eggs can stick to the tape. The tape is then examined under a microscope for the presence of eggs.

Note: This method is a recognized test often suggested by healthcare providers, particularly in pediatric cases, but it is not entirely "natural" as it involves an external tool (tape).

Coconut Oil Test

What It Is: Proponents suggest that ingesting coconut oil, which is believed to have antiparasitic properties, might help identify a parasitic infection based on the body's response.

How It's Done: Consume 1-2 tablespoons of raw, extra-virgin coconut oil daily and monitor for symptoms such as abdominal discomfort or changes in bowel movements, which some believe could indicate a parasitic presence.

Note: As with garlic, any symptoms experienced could be due to various factors, including a reaction to the oil itself, rather than an indication of parasites.

Herbal Remedy Response

What It Is: This approach involves using specific herbs known for their antiparasitic properties and observing any die-off symptoms or changes in health.

How It's Done: Commonly used herbs include wormwood, black walnut hull, and cloves. These are taken as supplements or teas, and any die-off reaction (like fatigue, headaches, or digestive changes) is considered by some as an indication of a parasitic infection.

Note: Reactions can also be due to the potency of the herbs or personal sensitivities and are not a reliable diagnostic method.

These natural tests are largely based on anecdotal evidence and are not substitutes for proper medical diagnosis. If you suspect a parasitic infection, it is crucial to consult a healthcare professional for accurate testing and diagnosis. Traditional medical diagnostics, such as stool tests, blood tests, and imaging, remain the most reliable methods for detecting parasitic infections.

CONVENTIONAL DIAGNOSTIC METHODS

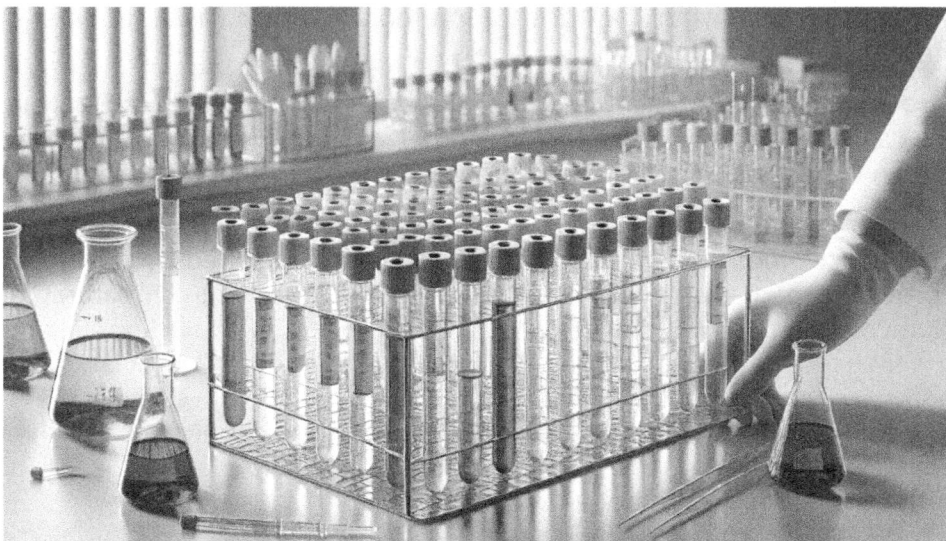

For a more accurate and reliable diagnosis of parasitic infections, several conventional medical tests are employed:

Stool Examination

This common method analyzes a stool sample under a microscope to detect eggs, larvae, or adult parasites. It is particularly useful for diagnosing intestinal parasites like Giardia, Entamoeba histolytica, and various worms. Multiple samples may be required to improve detection accuracy.

Blood Tests

Blood tests detect parasites that reside in the bloodstream or identify antibodies produced in response to an infection. For example, blood smears can reveal malaria parasites, while serological tests can detect antibodies for Toxoplasma gondii or Trichinella spiralis.

Imaging Techniques

Ultrasound, X-rays, CT scans, and MRI are used to detect parasitic infections affecting internal organs. These methods are effective for identifying cysts caused by parasites like Echinococcus granulosus in the liver or lungs, or neurocysticercosis in the brain.

Endoscopy and Colonoscopy

These procedures allow direct visualization of the gastrointestinal tract to diagnose parasitic infections. They can reveal lesions, ulcers, or the parasites themselves, such as tapeworms or hookworms, in the intestines.

Skin Biopsy

A small sample of skin is taken and examined under a microscope to identify parasites like mites causing scabies or larvae of hookworms. This method is used when parasitic infections manifest with skin symptoms.

Urine Tests

Useful for diagnosing infections like schistosomiasis, urine tests detect eggs of Schistosoma haematobium. This is particularly effective in regions where schistosomiasis is prevalent.

Serological Tests

These tests detect antibodies or antigens in the blood, indicating a parasitic infection. Examples include ELISA and IHA, which are used for diagnosing conditions such as toxoplasmosis and amoebiasis.

PCR (Polymerase Chain Reaction)

A highly sensitive molecular technique that amplifies DNA sequences to detect even minute amounts of parasitic DNA in various sample types, including blood and stool. It is particularly useful for diagnosing infections like malaria and toxoplasmosis.

Microscopic Examination

A fundamental diagnostic tool, microscopic examination involves looking at blood smears or stool samples to identify parasites directly. Skilled technicians can differentiate species based on their appearance, aiding accurate diagnosis and treatment.

Rapid Diagnostic Tests (RDTs)

RDTs provide quick and easy-to-use diagnostic options for certain parasitic infections, especially in resource-limited settings. These tests often involve dipsticks or cassettes that detect specific antigens or antibodies. RDTs are commonly used for malaria, with results available in minutes, facilitating timely treatment decisions.

Histopathology

Histopathology involves examining tissue samples under a microscope to identify parasitic infections. This method is particularly useful for diagnosing tissue-invasive parasites like Leishmania, Toxoplasma gondii, and Echinococcus. Histopathological examination can reveal the presence of parasites, cysts, or characteristic tissue reactions, aiding in diagnosis and treatment planning.

Clinical Presentation and History

A comprehensive patient history and clinical examination are vital for diagnosing parasitic infections. Healthcare providers consider travel history, exposure risks, and symptoms to identify potential infections.

Accurate diagnosis often requires a combination of these methods. Early detection and timely intervention are crucial to prevent complications and ensure effective treatment. If you suspect a parasitic infection, consider both natural indicators and conventional diagnostic tests to guide your approach.

Conclusion

Parasites, though often overlooked, represent a significant threat to human health globally. Their ability to adapt and thrive within their hosts makes them particularly challenging to detect and eradicate. Through this chapter, we have explored the diverse world of parasites, including protozoa, ectoparasites, and endoparasites, each with unique characteristics and life cycles.

Recognizing the common symptoms of parasitic infections, from gastrointestinal issues to neurological disturbances, is critical for early detection and intervention. The diagnostic methods discussed, ranging from stool examinations to advanced imaging techniques, underscore the importance of a comprehensive approach to identifying and managing these infections.

The journey to understanding parasites is both fascinating and essential. Armed with this knowledge, individuals can take proactive steps to protect their health, implement effective prevention strategies, and seek timely medical advice when necessary. This chapter serves as a foundation, providing the tools needed to navigate the complex landscape of parasitic infections and ultimately fostering a healthier, parasite-free life.

4. Preparing for Parasite Cleanse

Preparing for a parasite cleanse is a commendable step towards enhancing your overall health and well-being. However, preparation is key to ensuring a successful and safe cleanse. Chapter 4 delves into the essential steps you need to take before starting your cleanse. These preparations not only enhance the effectiveness of the cleanse but also help mitigate potential risks and ensure that your body is well-equipped to handle the detoxification process.

The first step in preparing for a parasite cleanse is assessing your personal health. This involves a thorough self-assessment to understand your current health status and mental preparation to brace yourself for the changes and challenges that lie ahead. Equally important is consulting with a healthcare professional, especially if you have underlying health conditions or are taking any medications. Their guidance can help tailor the cleanse to your specific needs, ensuring that it complements rather than conflicts with your health regimen.

Diet and nutrition play a crucial role in the success of your cleanse. A pre-cleanse diet helps to create an internal environment that is hostile to parasites and supportive of your body's natural detoxification processes. Understanding which foods to avoid and which ones to embrace can make a significant difference in the outcomes of your cleanse.

Finally, evaluating risks and taking necessary precautions cannot be overstated. This involves understanding the potential risks of natural cleanse methods, identifying contraindications for pre-existing health conditions, knowing when to consult a healthcare professional, and being aware of interactions with medications and other treatments. By thoroughly preparing for your cleanse, you can ensure that you approach this process with confidence, knowledge, and the necessary safeguards in place.

ASSESSING PERSONAL HEALTH

Starting a parasite cleanse is an important step in regaining your health and well-being. However, before beginning the cleanse, it's essential to thoroughly evaluate your health. This process includes self-assessment, mental preparation, and consulting with a healthcare professional to ensure the methods are safe and tailored to your specific health needs.

Self-Assessment and Mental Preparation

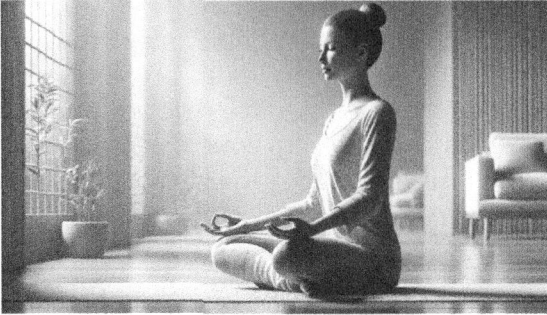

The path to a successful parasite cleanse starts with a thorough self-assessment. Understanding your body's current condition is essential for tailoring the cleanse to your specific needs. Begin by evaluating your overall health, paying attention to any symptoms that may indicate a parasitic infection, such as chronic fatigue, digestive issues, unexplained weight loss, or skin problems. Keep a detailed journal of your symptoms, noting their frequency and intensity, which will be valuable for consultations with health professionals.

Mental preparation is just as crucial. The idea of parasites in your body can be unsettling, and the cleansing process might bring mixed emotions. Cultivating a positive mindset is key. Educate yourself about parasites and the benefits of a natural cleanse to reduce fear and empower yourself. Visualize the end goal of a healthier, parasite-free body, and use mindfulness practices like meditation and deep breathing to stay calm and focused.

Understanding your motivations is another important aspect of mental preparation. Reflect on why you want to cleanse—whether to boost energy, resolve digestive issues, or enhance overall well-being. Clear motivations will help you stay committed, even during challenging phases of the cleanse. Sharing your goals with supportive friends or family can provide encouragement and accountability.

Finally, prepare your environment. Ensure your home is stocked with necessary supplies like herbs, supplements, and clean water. Organize your schedule to include time for relaxation and self-care. This holistic approach—combining physical, mental, and environmental preparation—lays the foundation for a successful parasite cleanse.

Consultation with a Healthcare Professional

While self-assessment and mental preparation are crucial, consulting a healthcare professional is a wise next step. This ensures that your cleanse methods align with your overall health and don't interfere with existing treatments or medications. Seek out experts in natural health, such as integrative doctors, naturopaths, or holistic health coaches. They can offer personalized advice, adjust your cleanse to fit your health needs, and monitor your progress to minimize risks.

During your consultation, share your detailed symptom journal, and be transparent about your health history, current medications, and past cleansing experiences. This openness allows the professional to provide the best possible guidance. They may recommend specific tests to confirm a parasitic infection or identify conditions that could impact your cleanse.

While this book emphasizes natural methods, it's important to recognize that some situations may require conventional medical treatment. If your symptoms worsen or new severe symptoms emerge, seek immediate medical attention. Balancing natural and medical approaches ensures a safe and effective cleanse.

In summary, combining thorough self-assessment and mental preparation with professional guidance is key to a successful parasite cleanse. By understanding your body, preparing your mind, and consulting with knowledgeable professionals, you lay a strong foundation for a transformative and health-boosting cleanse.

PRE-CLEANSE DIET AND NUTRITION

Starting a parasite cleanse is a key move toward restoring your health and vitality. An essential part of this process is modifying your diet to support the cleanse. A pre-cleanse diet is crucial for two main reasons: it readies your body for detoxification and helps create an internal environment that discourages parasites. This section will cover which foods to avoid and which ones enhance the effectiveness of your cleanse.

Foods to Avoid

Understanding which foods to eliminate from your diet is crucial in minimizing the conditions that allow parasites to thrive. Here are key categories of foods to avoid:

Sugary Foods: Sugar is a primary food source for many parasites. High sugar intake can create an environment conducive to parasitic growth and reproduction. This includes not only obvious sources like candies, pastries, and sugary drinks but also hidden sugars found in processed foods. Even natural sugars in fruits should be consumed in moderation during the cleanse. High glycemic fruits such as bananas, grapes, and mangoes can spike blood sugar levels, providing nourishment for parasites.

Refined Carbohydrates: Refined carbs, such as white bread, pasta, and pastries, quickly convert into sugars in the body, providing sustenance for parasites. These foods lack the fiber necessary to support healthy digestion and can contribute to constipation, further complicating the cleansing process.

Dairy Products: Dairy can be difficult to digest for many people and can lead to mucus production, which may create a hospitable environment for parasites. Furthermore, lactose in dairy products can feed certain types of parasites. It's advisable to reduce or eliminate milk, cheese, and yogurt from your diet during the cleanse.

Processed Foods: Foods high in preservatives, artificial colors, and additives can burden your liver and hinder the detoxification process. These foods often lack the nutrients needed to support your immune system and digestive health, making it harder for your body to fight off parasites.

Alcohol and Caffeine: Alcohol can weaken your immune system and impair liver function, both of which are critical in the fight against parasites. Caffeine, on the other hand, can dehydrate the body and over-stimulate the nervous system, making it harder to relax and allow the body to heal.

Foods that Support Parasite Cleanse

While avoiding certain foods is essential, equally important is incorporating foods that support your body's natural defenses and aid in the elimination of parasites. Here are some of the most effective foods to include in your pre-cleanse diet:

Garlic: Garlic is renowned for its potent antimicrobial properties. It contains sulfur compounds that are effective against a variety of parasites. Consuming raw garlic can help kill parasites and prevent their growth. Adding crushed garlic to your salads or smoothies can provide an added boost to your cleanse.

Pumpkin Seeds: Pumpkin seeds are rich in cucurbitacin, a compound that paralyzes parasites, making them easier to expel from the body. Consuming a handful of raw pumpkin seeds daily can support your cleanse by directly targeting intestinal parasites.

Papaya Seeds: Papaya seeds have been used traditionally to combat parasites. They contain enzymes like papain that can help break down protein walls of parasites. Blending a few papaya seeds into a smoothie can be an effective way to harness their benefits.

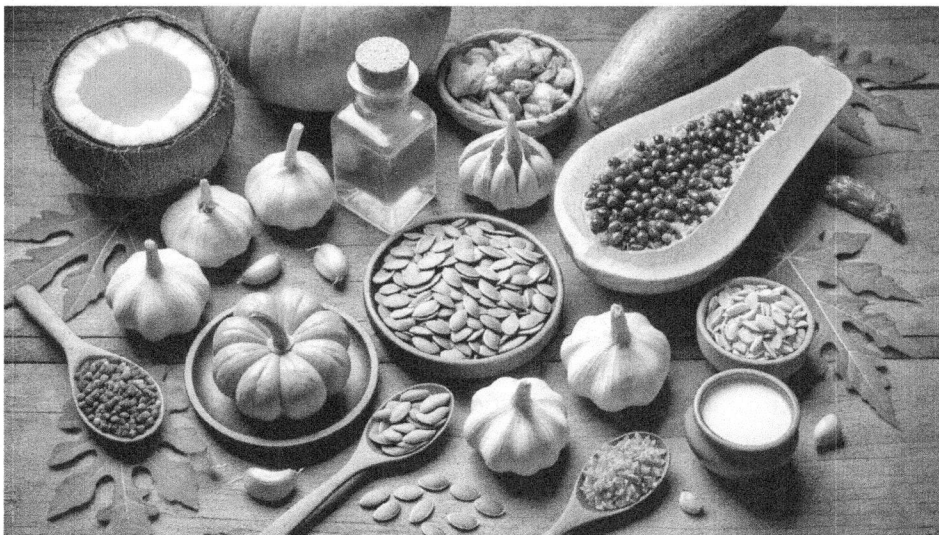

Coconut Oil: Coconut oil is rich in medium-chain fatty acids, particularly lauric acid, which has antiparasitic properties. Incorporating coconut oil into your diet can help eliminate parasites while also providing a source of healthy fats. You can use it in cooking or add a spoonful to your morning coffee or smoothie.

Pineapple: Pineapple contains bromelain, an enzyme that can help break down parasites and their eggs. Fresh pineapple, as opposed to canned or processed, is most effective. Consuming a few slices of pineapple daily can aid in the digestive process and support the elimination of parasites.

Turmeric: Turmeric is a powerful anti-inflammatory and antimicrobial spice. Its active compound, curcumin, has been shown to be effective against a range of parasites. Adding turmeric to your meals or consuming it as a tea can help support your cleanse.

Ginger: Ginger is another potent antimicrobial that aids digestion and helps expel parasites. Fresh ginger can be added to teas, smoothies, or meals to harness its benefits. Ginger also helps reduce inflammation and can soothe digestive discomfort.

Carrots: Carrots are rich in beta-carotene, which the body converts to vitamin A. This vitamin is essential for a strong immune system and can help the body fight off parasitic infections. Eating raw carrots as a snack or adding them to salads and smoothies can support your cleanse.

Apple Cider Vinegar: Apple cider vinegar (ACV) helps to alkalize the body and create an inhospitable environment for parasites. Diluting ACV in water and drinking it before meals can improve digestion and support detoxification. The acetic acid in ACV can help kill parasites and support the body's natural cleansing processes.

Green Leafy Vegetables: Leafy greens such as spinach, kale, and arugula are rich in nutrients and fiber, aiding in the detoxification process. These vegetables support liver function and provide essential vitamins and minerals that strengthen the immune system. Incorporating a variety of greens in salads, smoothies, and meals is highly beneficial.

Probiotic-Rich Foods: Foods like sauerkraut, kimchi, kefir, and kombucha are rich in probiotics, which support a healthy gut microbiome. A balanced gut flora can help keep parasites in check and improve overall digestive health. Including these foods in your diet can help maintain a healthy internal environment.

Herbal Teas: Herbal teas such as peppermint, chamomile, and dandelion root can support digestion and liver function. These teas can also have mild antiparasitic properties and help soothe the digestive tract. Drinking herbal teas regularly can be a gentle yet effective way to support your cleanse.

Fermented Foods: Fermented foods such as yogurt, miso, and tempeh are also rich in beneficial bacteria. These foods can help repopulate the gut with healthy bacteria, making it less hospitable for parasites. Including a variety of fermented foods in your diet can enhance your body's natural defenses.

Berries: Berries such as blueberries, strawberries, and raspberries are high in antioxidants and fiber. These fruits can help support the immune system and provide a source of natural energy. Berries can be consumed fresh or added to smoothies and salads.

Water: Staying hydrated is crucial during a parasite cleanse. Water helps flush out toxins and supports all bodily functions. Aim to drink at least eight glasses of water a day, and consider adding a slice of lemon or lime for added detox benefits.

By adjusting your diet to include these supportive foods and eliminate those that hinder your progress, you set the stage for a successful parasite cleanse. Your body will be better equipped to expel parasites, reduce inflammation, and restore balance. This dietary foundation not only aids in the immediate cleanse but also promotes long-term health and resilience against future parasitic infections.

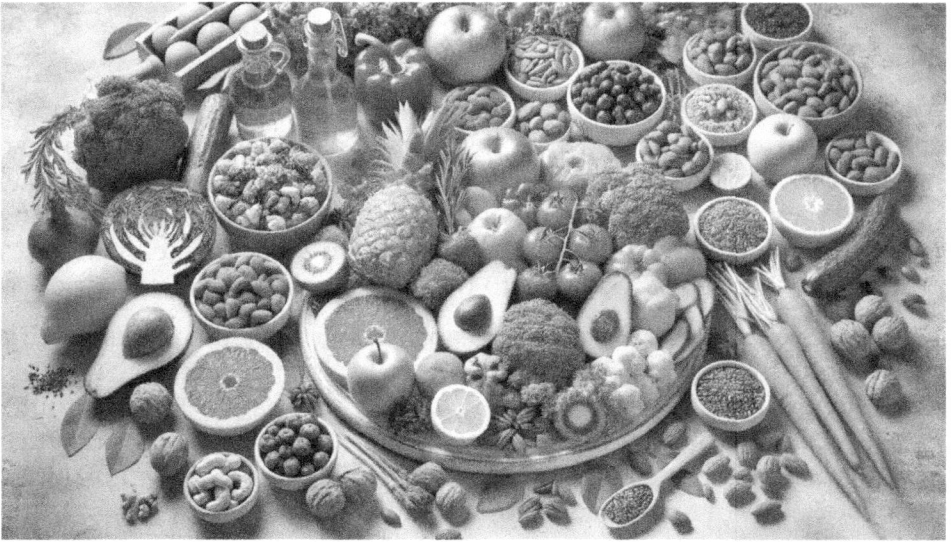

EVALUATING RISKS AND PRECAUTIONS

A parasite cleanse can significantly improve your health, but it's crucial to understand the potential risks and precautions of natural methods. Being aware of these factors will help you navigate the process safely and effectively, maximizing benefits while minimizing adverse effects. This knowledge ensures a more successful and comfortable cleansing experience.

Potential Risks of Natural Cleanse Methods

Natural parasite cleanse methods, while generally safe, are not entirely without risk. It's crucial to understand these risks to make informed decisions throughout your cleanse journey.

Herxheimer Reaction: The Herxheimer reaction, or "die-off" reaction, occurs when parasites die rapidly and release toxins into the body. This can lead to symptoms such as headaches, nausea, flu-like symptoms, and fatigue. While this reaction indicates that the cleanse is working, it can be uncomfortable and alarming. Staying well-hydrated, resting, and supporting your body with nutrient-rich foods can help manage these symptoms.

Digestive Disturbances: Natural cleanse methods often involve substances that can disrupt the digestive system. Herbs like wormwood and black walnut, though effective, can cause gastrointestinal discomfort, including cramping, diarrhea, and bloating. It's important to start with lower doses and gradually increase them to allow your body to adjust.

Listening to your body and adjusting the dosage as needed is key to minimizing these side effects.

Allergic Reactions: Some individuals may have allergic reactions to certain herbs or supplements used in a parasite cleanse. Symptoms can range from mild, such as itching and rashes, to severe, including difficulty breathing and anaphylaxis. Before starting any new herb or supplement, it's wise to conduct a patch test or consult with a healthcare provider to ensure you do not have allergies to the ingredients.

Nutrient Depletion: Aggressive cleansing can sometimes lead to the depletion of essential nutrients in the body. For instance, certain detoxifying agents may also bind to vitamins and minerals, causing their excretion. To counter this, ensure you are consuming a balanced diet rich in nutrients and consider taking a multivitamin supplement to maintain adequate levels of essential vitamins and minerals.

Contraindications for Pre-Existing Health Conditions

Individuals with certain pre-existing health conditions should approach natural parasite cleanse methods with caution. Here are some specific considerations:

Pregnancy and Breastfeeding: Pregnant or breastfeeding women should avoid many cleansing herbs and supplements, as they can affect the fetus or infant. Ingredients like wormwood and black walnut hull are not recommended during pregnancy due to their potential to cause uterine contractions or other adverse effects. Consulting a healthcare provider before starting any cleanse during these periods is crucial.

Autoimmune Disorders: For individuals with autoimmune disorders, certain cleanse methods might exacerbate their condition. Some herbs and supplements can stimulate the immune system, potentially leading to flare-ups. It's essential for individuals with autoimmune conditions to work closely with their healthcare provider to choose a safe and appropriate cleansing protocol.

Liver and Kidney Conditions: People with liver or kidney conditions need to be particularly cautious, as these organs play a significant role in detoxification. Some natural cleanse methods can put additional strain on the liver and kidneys, potentially worsening these conditions. Monitoring liver and kidney function and seeking medical advice before starting a cleanse is advisable for these individuals.

Chronic Illnesses: Individuals with chronic illnesses such as diabetes, heart disease, or severe gastrointestinal disorders should also exercise caution. Cleansing can impact blood sugar levels, electrolyte balance, and overall stability. It's vital to tailor the cleanse to individual needs and closely monitor any changes in symptoms or health status.

When to Consult a Healthcare Professional

Consulting a healthcare professional is a prudent step before embarking on a parasite cleanse, especially if you have any pre-existing health conditions or concerns. Here are some scenarios where professional guidance is particularly important:

Uncertain Diagnosis: If you suspect a parasitic infection but are unsure, a healthcare provider can help with accurate diagnosis and appropriate treatment recommendations. They can conduct tests to identify specific parasites and tailor the cleanse accordingly.

Severe Symptoms: Experiencing severe or worsening symptoms during a cleanse warrants immediate medical attention. Symptoms like extreme abdominal pain, persistent vomiting, or severe allergic reactions should not be ignored. A healthcare provider can help assess the situation and provide necessary interventions.

Medication Interactions: If you are on prescription medications, it's crucial to consult a healthcare professional to ensure there are no harmful interactions with the herbs and supplements used in the cleanse. Some natural ingredients can interfere with the effectiveness or increase the side effects of medications.

Customized Cleanse Plans: For individuals with complex health histories or multiple conditions, a healthcare provider can help develop a customized cleanse plan that considers all aspects of their health. This personalized approach can enhance safety and efficacy.

Interactions with Medications and Other Treatments

Understanding potential interactions between natural cleanse methods and existing medications or treatments is vital to avoid adverse effects. Here are some key considerations:

Anticoagulants: Herbs like garlic and ginger, commonly used in parasite cleanses, have blood-thinning properties. If you are taking anticoagulant medications such as warfarin, combining them with these herbs can increase the risk of bleeding. It's essential to monitor blood clotting parameters and consult a healthcare provider to adjust dosages appropriately.

Immunosuppressants: Individuals on immunosuppressant medications, such as those prescribed after organ transplants or for autoimmune diseases, need to be cautious. Some herbs can stimulate the immune system, potentially counteracting the effects of immunosuppressants. Close monitoring and consultation with a healthcare provider are necessary to balance the effects.

Diabetes Medications: Certain cleanse ingredients can affect blood sugar levels. For individuals taking insulin or other diabetes medications, herbs like cinnamon and berberine, which can lower blood sugar, may require adjustments in medication dosages. Regular blood sugar monitoring and healthcare provider consultations are crucial.

Antibiotics: Taking antibiotics alongside a parasite cleanse can be counterproductive. Some natural cleanse methods can interfere with the absorption or effectiveness of antibiotics. It's advisable to complete antibiotic courses before starting a cleanse or to separate the timing of doses significantly.

Thyroid Medications: Ingredients like kelp and iodine supplements used in cleanses can affect thyroid function. For individuals on thyroid medications, these ingredients can either enhance or diminish the medication's effects. Regular thyroid function tests and healthcare provider guidance are essential in such cases.

By carefully evaluating risks and taking necessary precautions, you can embark on your parasite cleanse journey with confidence. Understanding the potential interactions and seeking professional guidance when needed ensures that your cleanse is both safe and effective. This comprehensive approach not only supports the elimination of parasites but also promotes overall health and well-being.

Conclusion

Preparing for a parasite cleanse involves more than just gathering supplies. It requires a comprehensive approach that includes assessing your physical and mental health for a more effective cleanse. Adjusting your diet and nutrition is essential to support detoxification and create an unfavorable environment for parasites. Equally important is evaluating potential risks and precautions to navigate the cleanse safely and minimize discomfort. This thorough preparation ensures you're not only ready to begin but also set up to achieve optimal results.

5. Introduction Natural Parasite Cleanse Methods

Natural parasite cleansing methods have been used for centuries, drawing on the healing power of plants and traditional practices to combat parasitic infections. In this chapter, we explore a variety of herbs and supplements known for their antiparasitic properties, as well as other natural methods that have gained popularity in recent years. Our goal is to provide you with a comprehensive guide to the most effective natural remedies available, allowing you to choose the best approach for your health needs.

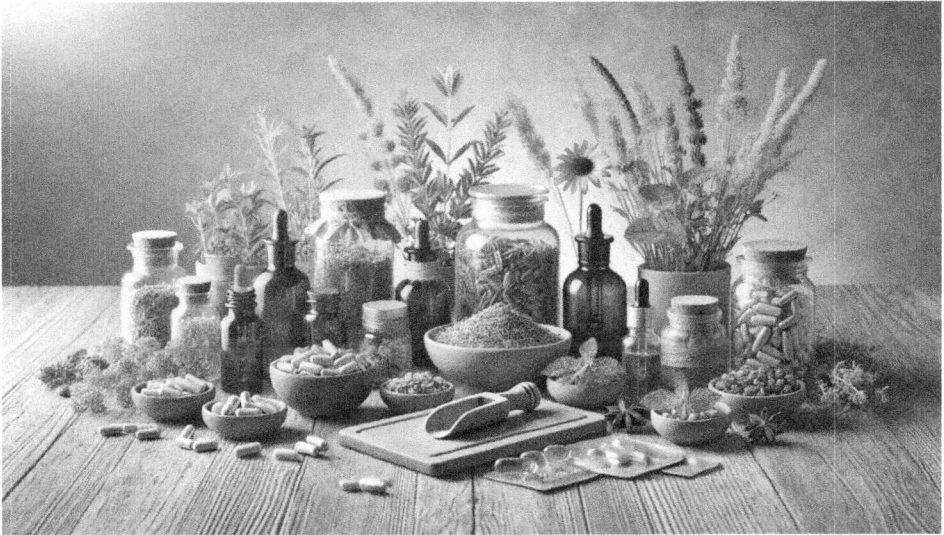

Herbs and supplements such as aloe vera, black walnut, garlic, and turmeric are renowned for their ability to support the body in eliminating parasites and improving overall wellness. Each of these natural remedies offers unique benefits, from boosting the immune system to directly targeting parasitic organisms. By understanding the properties and uses of these herbs, you can develop a personalized parasite cleanse regimen that aligns with your health goals.

In addition to herbs and supplements, we also delve into other natural methods such as oil pulling with coconut oil, coffee enemas, and bentonite clay. While these techniques can offer additional support in a parasite cleanse, it is essential to approach them with caution and under the guidance of a healthcare professional. Some of these methods carry significant risks if not used correctly, and it is crucial to prioritize safety in your health journey.

As you read through this chapter, you'll gain insights into the function, characteristics, and recommended usage of each herb and method. Our aim is to empower you with the knowledge needed to make informed decisions about your health and to explore natural remedies confidently and safely. By integrating these practices into your lifestyle, you can enhance your well-being and take proactive steps toward a parasite-free body.

HERBS AND SUPPLEMENTS

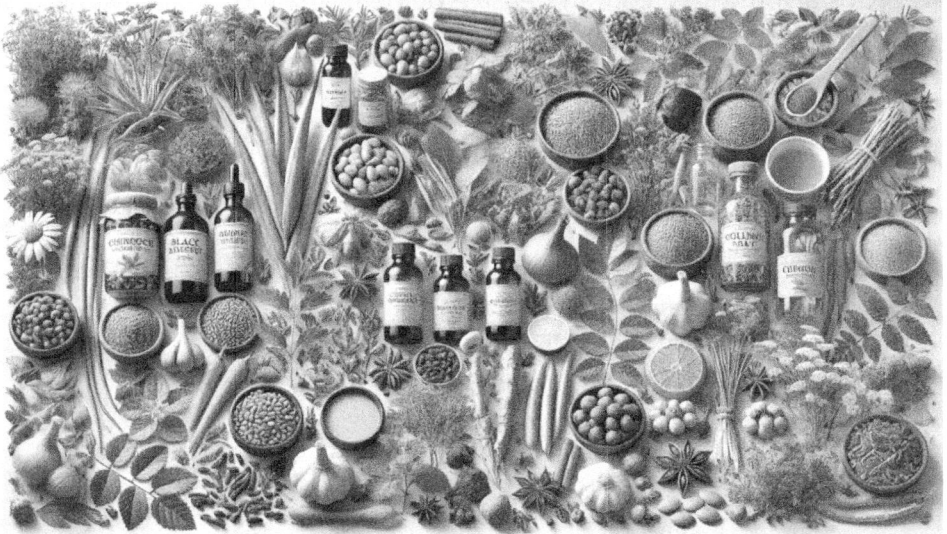

Aloe Vera

Aloe Vera, known for its thick, fleshy leaves, contains a gel rich in vitamins, minerals, and amino acids. This gel is renowned for its soothing and healing properties, particularly for the digestive tract. Aloe Vera aids in cleansing the gut by promoting bowel movements and supporting the elimination of waste. Its anti-inflammatory and antimicrobial properties make it effective against certain parasites. To use, extract the gel from the leaves and consume it directly or mix it with water or juice. Recommended dose: 1-2 tablespoons of fresh gel daily.

Anise

Anise, with its sweet, licorice-like flavor, has been used for centuries to treat digestive issues. The seeds contain anethole, which has antifungal, antibacterial, and antiparasitic properties. Anise helps expel intestinal worms and reduces bloating and discomfort. It is typically consumed as a tea, made by steeping crushed anise seeds in hot water, or added to dishes as a spice. Recommended dose: 1-2 cups of anise tea daily.

Barberry

Barberry, a shrub with bright red berries, contains berberine, a compound known for its antimicrobial properties. Berberine is effective against various parasites, bacteria, and fungi. Barberry helps cleanse the liver, improve digestion, and support the immune system. The berries or root bark can be used to make tea, or berberine supplements can be taken directly. Recommended dose: 500 mg of berberine supplement daily or 1-2 cups of barberry tea.

Berberine

Berberine, found in plants like goldenseal, barberry, and Oregon grape, is a powerful alkaloid with broad-spectrum antimicrobial activity. It disrupts the cellular structure of parasites, making it an effective natural remedy for eliminating them. Berberine also supports gut health by balancing the microbiome and reducing inflammation. Commonly available in supplement form, it should be taken according to recommended dosages. Recommended dose: 500-1500 mg daily, divided into 2-3 doses.

Black Walnut Hull

Black Walnut hulls contain juglone, tannins, and iodine, which have potent antiparasitic properties. They are highly effective against intestinal worms, including tapeworms and pinworms. The hulls are often ground into a powder or made into a tincture. Black Walnut hull is particularly effective when combined with wormwood and cloves in a parasite cleanse protocol. Recommended dose: 2-4 ml of tincture or 500 mg of powdered hulls daily.

Burdock Root

Burdock Root is known for its blood-purifying properties, helping to detoxify the body and support the liver. It has antimicrobial and antiparasitic effects, making it valuable for a cleanse. Burdock Root can be consumed as a tea, tincture, or added to soups and stews. Recommended dose: 1-2 cups of burdock root tea daily or 1-2 ml of tincture.

Castor Oil

Castor Oil, derived from the seeds of the castor plant, is a powerful laxative that helps expel parasites and their waste from the intestines. It also has anti-inflammatory properties and supports overall gut health. Castor Oil should be used with caution and under guidance, as it is a strong purgative. Recommended dose: 1-2 teaspoons taken with warm water, used only occasionally.

Cayenne Pepper

Cayenne Pepper, known for its spicy kick, contains capsaicin, which has powerful antimicrobial properties. It helps increase circulation, stimulate digestion, and expel parasites from the digestive tract. Cayenne Pepper can be added to foods, taken as a supplement, or mixed with water and lemon for a cleansing drink. Recommended dose: 1/4 teaspoon in food or drink daily.

Chamomile

Chamomile is a gentle herb with calming properties that soothes the digestive tract and reduces inflammation. It also has mild antiparasitic effects and supports the body during a cleanse by promoting relaxation and reducing stress. Chamomile is best consumed as a tea, made by steeping the dried flowers in hot water. Recommended dose: 1-2 cups of chamomile tea daily.

Chlorophyll

Chlorophyll, the green pigment found in plants, helps detoxify the body and promote healing. It supports gut health and eliminates parasites by oxygenating the blood and tissues. Chlorophyll supplements are available in liquid or capsule form and can be taken daily to support a cleanse. Recommended dose: 1-2 teaspoons of liquid chlorophyll or 100-300 mg in capsule form daily.

Cilantro (Coriander)

Cilantro is a potent herb for detoxification, particularly for heavy metals and parasites. It binds to toxins and helps expel them from the body. Cilantro can be added to salads, smoothies, and dishes, or taken as a juice or extract for a more concentrated effect. Recommended dose: A handful of fresh cilantro daily or 1-2 ml of extract.

Cloves

Cloves contain eugenol, a powerful compound with antiparasitic properties. They are particularly effective against parasite eggs, helping break the life cycle and prevent reinfestation. Cloves can be consumed as a tea, taken in capsule form, or added to dishes as a spice. Recommended dose: 1-2 cups of clove tea or 500 mg of clove capsules daily.

Coconut Oil

Coconut Oil is rich in medium-chain fatty acids, particularly lauric acid, which has strong antimicrobial and antiparasitic effects. It helps dissolve the protective membranes of parasites, making them easier to eliminate. Coconut Oil can be consumed directly, used in cooking, or taken as part of an oil pulling regimen. Recommended dose: 1-2 tablespoons daily.

Diatomaceous Earth

Diatomaceous Earth is a natural powder made from fossilized algae. It works by physically damaging the exoskeletons of parasites, leading to their death. It also helps cleanse the digestive tract and remove toxins. Food-grade Diatomaceous Earth can be mixed with water or juice and consumed daily during a cleanse. Recommended dose: 1 tablespoon mixed with water or juice daily.

Echinacea

Echinacea is well-known for its immune-boosting properties and has antimicrobial effects that help fight parasitic infections. Echinacea can be taken as a tea, tincture, or supplement to support the immune system during a cleanse. Recommended dose: 1-2 cups of echinacea tea or 2-4 ml of tincture daily.

Epazote

Epazote is a traditional herb used in Mexican cuisine with strong antiparasitic properties, particularly effective against intestinal worms. Fresh or dried Epazote leaves can be added to soups, stews, and bean dishes. Recommended dose: A few fresh or dried leaves added to meals daily.

Fenugreek Seeds

Fenugreek Seeds have antimicrobial and anti-inflammatory properties that support gut health and help eliminate parasites. They aid digestion and soothe the digestive tract. Fenugreek Seeds can be soaked and added to salads, ground into powder, or taken as a supplement. Recommended dose: 1-2 teaspoons of seeds or 500 mg of powder daily.

Garlic

Garlic is one of the most potent natural antiparasitic foods. It contains allicin, a compound with strong antimicrobial properties that kill parasites and support overall health. Raw garlic can be added to dishes, consumed directly, or taken as a supplement. Recommended dose: 1-2 cloves of raw garlic daily or 600-900 mg of garlic extract.

Ginger

Ginger has powerful anti-inflammatory and antimicrobial properties that soothe the digestive tract, stimulate digestion, and eliminate parasites. Fresh ginger can be added to teas, smoothies, and dishes, or taken as a supplement. Recommended dose: 1-2 inches of fresh ginger or 500-1000 mg of ginger extract daily.

Goldenseal

Goldenseal contains berberine, which has broad-spectrum antimicrobial activity. It supports the digestive system and helps eliminate parasites. Goldenseal can be taken as a tea, tincture, or supplement, often in combination with other herbs like Echinacea. Recommended dose: 500-1000 mg of goldenseal extract or 2-4 ml of tincture daily.

Grapefruit Seed Extract

Grapefruit Seed Extract is a powerful antimicrobial agent that helps eliminate parasites. It disrupts the cell membranes of parasites and supports the immune system. The extract can be taken in liquid or capsule form. Recommended dose: 10-15 drops of liquid extract or 200-400 mg in capsule form daily.

Holy Basil (Tulsi)

Holy Basil, also known as Tulsi, has antimicrobial and anti-inflammatory properties. It supports the immune system and helps eliminate parasites. Holy Basil can be consumed as a tea, taken as a supplement, or used in cooking. Recommended dose: 1-2 cups of Tulsi tea or 400-800 mg of supplement daily.

Mimosa Pudica

Mimosa Pudica is a tropical plant with seeds that have strong antiparasitic properties. The seeds form a gel-like substance that traps and eliminates parasites. Mimosa Pudica seeds can be taken in capsule form as part of a cleanse protocol. Recommended dose: 2-4 capsules (500 mg each) daily.

Neem

Neem has been used for centuries in Ayurvedic medicine for its antimicrobial properties. It helps eliminate parasites and support the immune system. Neem leaves, oil, or extract can be used in various forms, including teas, tinctures, and supplements. Recommended dose: 1-2 teaspoons of neem powder or 300-600 mg of neem extract daily.

Olive Leaf Extract

Olive Leaf Extract contains oleuropein, a compound with strong antimicrobial and antiparasitic effects. It supports the immune system and helps eliminate parasites. Olive Leaf Extract can be taken in liquid or capsule form. Recommended dose: 500-1000 mg of extract daily.

Oregano

Oregano is rich in carvacrol and thymol, compounds with powerful antimicrobial properties. It helps eliminate parasites and support gut health. Oregano oil or dried oregano can be used in cooking or taken as a supplement. Recommended dose: 500-1000 mg of oregano oil or 1-2 teaspoons of dried oregano daily.

Papaya Seeds

Papaya Seeds contain enzymes like papain that have strong antiparasitic properties. They help digest and expel parasites from the digestive tract. Papaya seeds can be consumed raw, blended into smoothies, or dried and ground into powder. Recommended dose: 1-2 teaspoons of seeds or powder daily.

Pau d'Arco

Pau d'Arco is a tree bark with strong antimicrobial properties. It helps eliminate parasites and support the immune system. Pau d'Arco can be consumed as a tea or taken in supplement form. Recommended dose: 1-2 cups of tea or 500-1000 mg of supplement daily.

Probiotics

Probiotics help balance the gut microbiome and support the immune system. They can help prevent and eliminate parasitic infections by promoting healthy gut flora. Probiotics are available in supplement form or can be obtained from fermented foods like yogurt, kefir, and sauerkraut. Recommended dose: 10-20 billion CFUs daily.

Pumpkin Seeds

Pumpkin Seeds contain cucurbitacin, a compound with antiparasitic properties. They help paralyze and expel intestinal worms. Pumpkin seeds can be eaten raw, roasted, or ground into powder and added to smoothies or dishes. Recommended dose: 1/4 cup of seeds or 2 tablespoons of powder daily.

Quassia

Quassia is a bitter herb with strong antiparasitic properties. It helps eliminate intestinal worms and support digestive health. Quassia can be consumed as a tea or taken as a supplement. Recommended dose: 1-2 cups of tea or 500-1000 mg of supplement daily.

Senna

Senna is a natural laxative that helps cleanse the digestive tract and expel parasites. It should be used with caution and under guidance, as it can cause cramping and dehydration. Senna is commonly taken as a tea or in supplement form. Recommended dose: 1 cup of tea or 500 mg of supplement as needed.

Tansy

Tansy is a herb with strong antiparasitic properties. It helps eliminate intestinal worms and support digestive health. Tansy can be consumed as a tea or taken as a supplement but should be used with caution due to its potency. Recommended dose: 1 cup of tea or 300-600 mg of supplement daily.

Thyme

Thyme is rich in thymol, a compound with strong antimicrobial properties. It helps eliminate parasites and support gut health. Fresh or dried thyme can be used in cooking, or thyme oil can be taken as a supplement. Recommended dose: 1-2 teaspoons of dried thyme or 200-400 mg of thyme oil daily.

Turmeric

Turmeric contains curcumin, a compound with powerful anti-inflammatory and antimicrobial properties. It helps eliminate parasites and support overall health. Turmeric can be added to dishes, consumed as a tea, or taken as a supplement. Recommended dose: 1-2 teaspoons of turmeric powder or 500-1000 mg of curcumin extract daily.

Wormseed (Chenopodium)

Wormseed, also known as Chenopodium, has strong antiparasitic properties. It helps eliminate intestinal worms and support digestive health. Wormseed can be consumed as a tea or taken as a supplement, often in combination with other antiparasitic herbs. Recommended dose: 1 cup of tea or 500-1000 mg of supplement daily.

Wormwood

Wormwood is a potent herb known for its antiparasitic properties. It contains compounds like artemisinin that help eliminate parasites. Wormwood can be consumed as a tea, tincture, or taken in supplement form, often as part of a parasite cleanse protocol with black walnut hull and cloves. Recommended dose: 1-2 cups of tea or 500-1000 mg of supplement daily.

OTHER NATURAL METHODS

While there are numerous natural methods for parasite cleansing, it's crucial to approach these with caution. Some methods carry significant risks if not used correctly. Here is an overview of the most well-known methods, with a balanced discussion of their benefits and risks.

Oil Pulling with Coconut Oil

Oil pulling is an ancient practice that involves swishing coconut oil in the mouth for 15-20 minutes. It's believed to help remove toxins and parasites from the mouth and digestive system. While many find oil pulling beneficial for oral health, there is no definitive scientific evidence proving its effectiveness against parasites.

Benefits: Can improve oral health and reduce gum inflammation.

Risks: Generally safe, but should not be considered a substitute for proven antiparasitic treatments.

Coffee Enemas

Coffee enemas have been used for colon cleansing and stimulating the liver. While some advocates claim they can help remove parasites, this method carries significant risks, including electrolyte imbalances and rectal damage.

Benefits: May stimulate bile production and aid in liver detoxification.

Risks: Potential for electrolyte imbalances, infections, and rectal damage. Strongly discouraged without medical supervision.

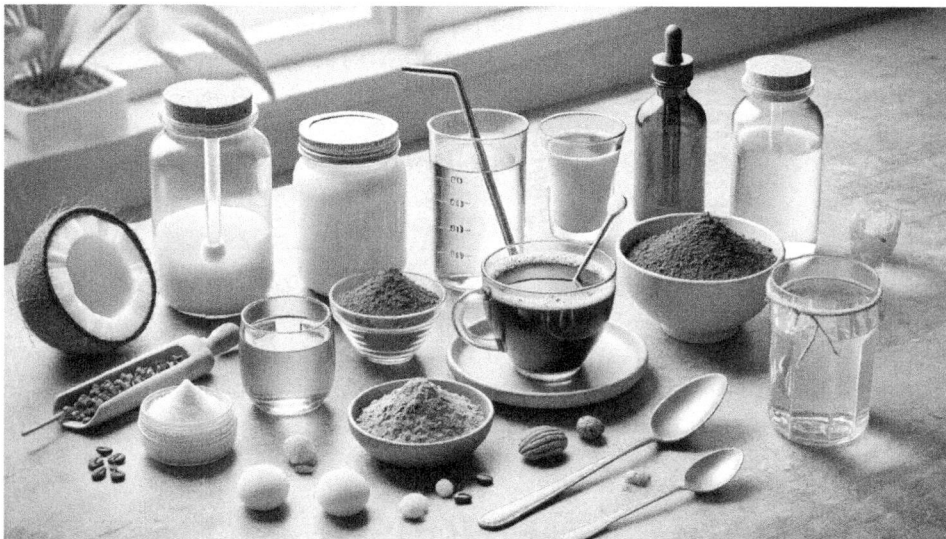

Bentonite Clay

Bentonite clay is a natural remedy believed to adsorb toxins and parasites from the digestive system. It can be taken internally or used externally in poultices.

Benefits: May help detoxify the body and improve digestive health.

Risks: Can cause constipation and, if not taken with adequate water, may lead to intestinal blockages. It's recommended to avoid internal use without professional guidance.

Colloidal Silver Water

Colloidal silver water is known for its antimicrobial properties. Some believe it can be effective against parasites, but there are concerns about the safety and side effects of taking colloidal silver.

Benefits: Strong antimicrobial properties.

Risks: Long-term use can lead to a condition called argyria, causing permanent blue-gray discoloration of the skin. Advised against for internal use due to potential health risks.

Water and Salt Cleansing

Water and salt cleansing involves drinking a saltwater solution to stimulate digestive cleansing. While it may effectively remove toxins, it can also pose risks if not done correctly.

Benefits: May help detoxify the digestive system.

Risks: Can cause dehydration and electrolyte imbalances. Should be approached with caution and ideally under professional supervision.

Conclusion

This chapter has delved into natural parasite cleansing methods, highlighting their advantages and potential drawbacks. We've explored how potent herbs and supplements like aloe vera, garlic, and turmeric can bolster overall health while combating parasites. Integrating these remedies into your daily regimen can fortify your body's innate defenses.

We've also addressed more controversial techniques such as coffee enemas and bentonite clay, emphasizing the need for caution due to associated risks. The importance of seeking professional medical advice before embarking on any new treatment regimen cannot be overstated.

Effective parasite cleansing hinges on a combination of informed decision-making, meticulous preparation, and expert guidance. By judiciously selecting appropriate herbs and supplements, and understanding the proper application of various methods, you can achieve a balanced, safe, and effective cleanse. This approach not only targets parasites but also prioritizes your overall well-being, paving the way for a healthier, parasite-free existence.

6. Parasite Cleanse Protocol

Incorporating a parasite cleanse into your routine can seem daunting, but with the right recipes and a structured program, it becomes a manageable and rewarding process. The goal of this chapter is to provide you with a comprehensive guide to recipes and a clear step-by-step program designed to support your body through the cleanse.

Understanding what you consume during this period is crucial. The recipes we've curated are not just delicious; they are packed with ingredients known for their anti-parasitic properties. From vibrant smoothies to hearty soups, these recipes will help create an environment in your body that is inhospitable to parasites while nourishing you deeply. Each ingredient has been carefully chosen for its unique benefits, ensuring that your cleanse is both effective and enjoyable.

The 30-day parasite cleanse program is designed to gradually prepare, cleanse, and restore your body. The first week focuses on preparation, helping your body to get ready for the intense phases that follow. Weeks two and three are the heart of the cleanse, where the focus is on eliminating parasites and supporting your body through this detoxification process. The final week is all about restoration, helping your body to heal and rebuild after the cleanse.

Moreover, maintaining these practices is key to long-term health. The maintenance program provides weekly, monthly, and seasonal strategies to keep your body parasite-free and functioning optimally. Flexibility is built into this program, allowing you to substitute recipes based on

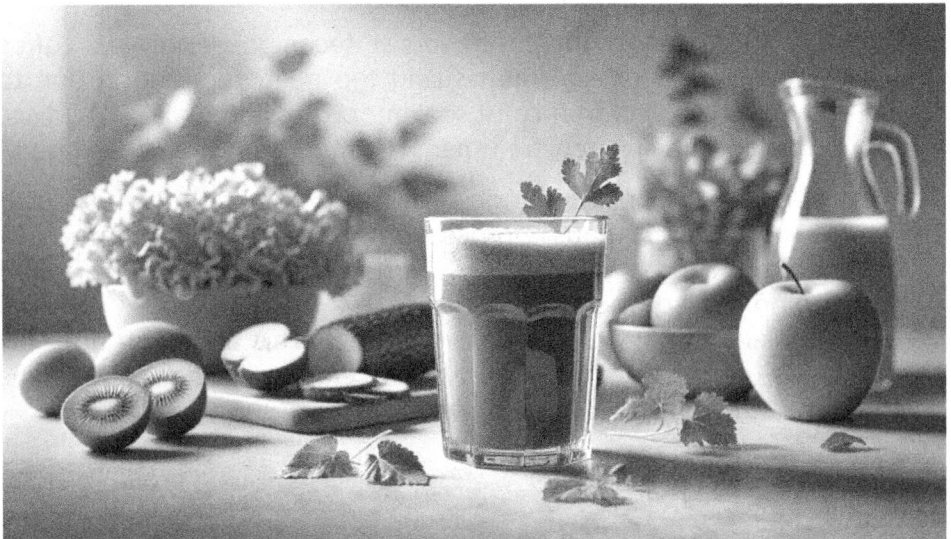

availability and personal preference while still adhering to the core principles of the cleanse. This approach ensures that the cleanse can fit seamlessly into your lifestyle, making it easier to follow and sustain over time.

RECIPES AND HOME REMEDIES

The journey to a parasite-free body can be greatly enhanced with the right dietary choices. Implementing specific recipes and home remedies into your daily routine can help eradicate parasites effectively and support overall health. Below, we explore various anti-parasitic juices, smoothies, soups, salads, herbal infusions, and more that are not only beneficial but also delicious.

Breakfast Recipes for the Parasite Cleanse

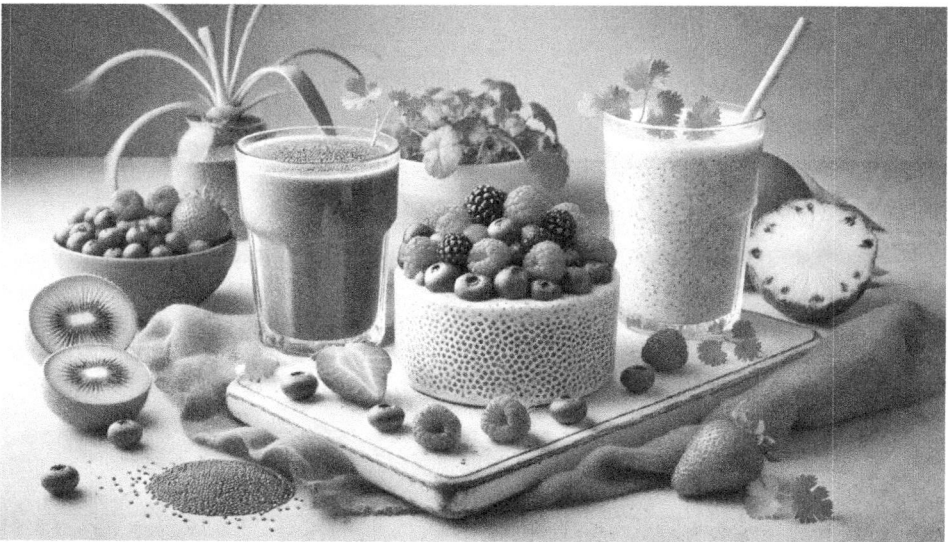

GREEN DETOX SMOOTHIE

Ingredients:	Directions:
<ul><li>1 cup spinach</li><li>1 cup kale</li><li>1/2 cucumber</li><li>1 green apple, cored</li><li>Juice of 1 lemon</li><li>1 cup water</li></ul>	<ul><li>Combine all ingredients in a blender.</li><li>Blend until smooth.</li><li>Drink immediately to get the most nutrients.</li></ul>

CILANTRO AND PINEAPPLE JUICE

Ingredients:	Directions:
<ul><li>1 cup fresh cilantro</li><li>1 cup pineapple chunks</li><li>1 cup water</li></ul>	<ul><li>Blend cilantro, pineapple, and water until smooth.</li><li>Strain the mixture to remove pulp (optional).</li><li>Drink immediately for a refreshing start to your day</li></ul>

PAPAYA SEED SMOOTHIE

Ingredients:	Directions:
<ul><li>1 tablespoon papaya seeds</li><li>1 cup papaya flesh, cubed</li><li>1 banana</li><li>1 cup coconut milk</li><li>1 teaspoon honey (optional)</li></ul>	<ul><li>Add papaya seeds, papaya flesh, banana, coconut milk, and honey to a blender.</li><li>Blend until smooth and creamy.</li><li>Drink immediately to enjoy the digestive benefits.</li></ul>

OVERNIGHT OATS WITH PUMPKIN SEEDS AND CINNAMON

Ingredients:	Directions:
<ul><li>1/2 cup rolled oats</li><li>1 cup almond milk</li><li>1 tablespoon pumpkin seeds</li><li>1/2 teaspoon cinnamon</li><li>1 tablespoon chia seeds</li><li>1 teaspoon honey or maple syrup (optional)</li></ul>	<ul><li>Combine all ingredients in a jar or bowl and mix well.</li><li>Cover and refrigerate overnight.</li><li>In the morning, stir and enjoy cold or warm slightly if preferred.</li></ul>

CHIA SEED PUDDING WITH FRESH BERRIES

Ingredients:	Directions:
<ul><li>3 tablespoons chia seeds</li><li>1 cup almond milk</li><li>1 teaspoon vanilla extract</li><li>1 tablespoon honey or maple syrup (optional)</li><li>1/2 cup fresh berries (strawberries, blueberries, raspberries)</li></ul>	<ul><li>In a bowl, mix chia seeds, almond milk, vanilla extract, and sweetener.</li><li>Stir well and refrigerate for at least 4 hours or overnight.</li><li>Top with fresh berries before serving.</li></ul>

ANTI-PARASITIC GRAIN BOWL

Ingredients:	Directions:
• 1/2 cup cooked quinoa or millet • 1/2 avocado, sliced • 1/4 cup sauerkraut or kimchi • 1 tablespoon pumpkin seeds • 1/2 cup mixed greens • 1 tablespoon olive oil • Juice of 1/2 lemon	• Assemble all ingredients in a bowl. • Drizzle with olive oil and lemon juice. • Enjoy a nourishing start to your day.

COCONUT OIL AND BERRY SMOOTHIE

Ingredients:	Directions:
• 1 cup mixed berries (strawberries, blueberries, raspberries) • 1 banana • 1 tablespoon coconut oil • 1 cup almond milk	• Blend all ingredients until smooth and creamy. • Drink immediately for a nutrient-packed breakfast.

SCRAMBLED EGGS WITH TURMERIC AND SPINACH

Ingredients:	Directions:
• 2 eggs • 1/2 teaspoon turmeric powder • 1 cup fresh spinach • 1 tablespoon coconut oil or olive oil • Salt and pepper to taste	• In a bowl, whisk the eggs with turmeric, salt, and pepper. • Heat oil in a skillet over medium heat. Add spinach and sauté until wilted. • Pour in the egg mixture and scramble until fully cooked. • Serve hot.

ANTI-PARASITIC CHIA PUDDING WITH COCONUT MILK

Ingredients:	Directions:
• 3 tablespoons chia seeds • 1 cup coconut milk • 1 tablespoon shredded coconut • 1 teaspoon honey or maple syrup (optional)	• Mix chia seeds, coconut milk, shredded coconut, and sweetener in a bowl. • Stir well and refrigerate for at least 4 hours or overnight. • Stir before eating and enjoy.

SPINACH AND AVOCADO TOAST

Ingredients:	Directions:
• 1 slice whole-grain bread, toasted • 1/2 avocado, mashed • 1/2 cup fresh spinach • 1 tablespoon pumpkin seeds • Salt, pepper, and red pepper flakes to taste	• Spread mashed avocado on toasted bread. • Top with fresh spinach and sprinkle with pumpkin seeds. • Season with salt, pepper, and red pepper flakes.

GREEN DETOX SMOOTHIE WITH SPIRULINA

Ingredients:	Directions:
• 1 cup spinach • 1/2 cucumber • 1 green apple, cored • 1/2 teaspoon spirulina powder • Juice of 1/2 lemon • 1 cup water	• Blend all ingredients until smooth. • Drink immediately for a nutrient boost.

ANTI-PARASITIC OVERNIGHT OATS WITH PUMPKIN SEEDS

Ingredients:	Directions:
• 1/2 cup rolled oats • 1 cup almond milk • 2 tablespoons pumpkin seeds • 1/2 teaspoon cinnamon • 1 tablespoon chia seeds • 1 teaspoon honey or maple syrup (optional)	• Combine oats, almond milk, pumpkin seeds, cinnamon, chia seeds, and sweetener in a jar or bowl. • Mix well, cover, and refrigerate overnight. • Stir and enjoy cold or warm slightly in the morning.

Lunch Recipes for the Parasite Cleanse

QUINOA AND AVOCADO SALAD

Ingredients:	Directions:
• 1 cup cooked quinoa • 1 avocado, diced • 1 cup cherry tomatoes, halved • 1 cucumber, diced • 1/4 cup red onion, finely chopped • 2 tablespoons olive oil • Juice of 1 lemon • Salt and pepper to taste	• In a large bowl, combine cooked quinoa, avocado, cherry tomatoes, cucumber, and red onion. • Drizzle with olive oil and lemon juice. • Season with salt and pepper, then toss gently to combine. • Serve fresh.

CHICKPEA SALAD WRAP

Ingredients:	Directions:
• 1 cup cooked chickpeas, mashed • 1/4 cup diced celery • 1/4 cup diced red bell pepper • 2 tablespoons tahini • Juice of 1 lemon • Salt and pepper to taste • 4 whole-grain wraps • Lettuce leaves	• In a bowl, mix together mashed chickpeas, celery, red bell pepper, tahini, lemon juice, salt, and pepper. • Spread the chickpea mixture onto each whole-grain wrap. • Add lettuce leaves and roll up tightly. • Cut in half and serve.

VEGETABLE STIR-FRY WITH TOFU

Ingredients:	Directions:
• 1 cup mixed vegetables (broccoli, bell peppers, carrots) • 1 cup tofu, diced • 1 tablespoon olive oil • 1 tablespoon soy sauce • 1 teaspoon grated ginger • 1 clove garlic, minced • 1/2 cup brown rice, cooked	• Heat olive oil in a skillet over medium heat. • Add garlic and ginger, sauté for 1 minute. • Add mixed vegetables and tofu, stir-fry until vegetables are tender and tofu is golden. • Stir in soy sauce. • Serve over cooked brown rice.

ROASTED PUMPKIN SEEDS AND MIXED GREEN SALAD

Ingredients:	Directions:
<ul><li>4 cups mixed greens</li><li>1/2 cup cherry tomatoes, halved</li><li>1/2 cucumber, diced</li><li>1/4 cup roasted pumpkin seeds</li><li>2 tablespoons olive oil</li><li>1 tablespoon balsamic vinegar</li><li>Salt and pepper to taste</li></ul>	<ul><li>In a large bowl, combine mixed greens, cherry tomatoes, cucumber, and roasted pumpkin seeds.</li><li>Drizzle with olive oil and balsamic vinegar.</li><li>Season with salt and pepper, then toss to combine.</li><li>Serve immediately.</li></ul>

FERMENTED VEGETABLE SALAD

Ingredients:	Directions:
<ul><li>1 cup sauerkraut</li><li>1 cup kimchi</li><li>4 cups mixed greens</li><li>2 tablespoons light vinaigrette</li></ul>	<ul><li>In a bowl, combine sauerkraut, kimchi, and mixed greens.</li><li>Drizzle with light vinaigrette and toss well.</li><li>Serve immediately for a tangy and probiotic-rich salad.</li></ul>

PUMPKIN SEED PESTO SALAD

Ingredients:	Directions:
<ul><li>4 cups mixed greens</li><li>1 cup cherry tomatoes, halved</li><li>1 cucumber, diced</li><li>1/2 cup pumpkin seed pesto (see recipe below)</li></ul>	<ul><li>Toss mixed greens with pumpkin seed pesto.</li><li>Top with cherry tomatoes and cucumber.</li><li>Serve fresh for a flavorful, nutrient-packed meal.</li></ul>

PUMPKIN SEED PESTO PASTA

Ingredients:	Directions:
<ul><li>8 oz whole-grain pasta</li><li>1/2 cup pumpkin seed pesto (see recipe below)</li><li>1 cup cherry tomatoes, halved</li><li>1/4 cup grated Parmesan cheese (optional)</li></ul>	<ul><li>Cook pasta according to package instructions. Drain and return to pot.</li><li>Add pumpkin seed pesto and cherry tomatoes to pasta, tossing to coat.</li><li>Sprinkle with Parmesan cheese, if using.</li><li>Serve warm.</li></ul>

SPINACH AND MUSHROOM QUINOA BOWL

Ingredients:	Directions:
<ul><li>1 cup cooked quinoa</li><li>1 cup sliced mushrooms</li><li>2 cups fresh spinach</li><li>1 tablespoon olive oil</li><li>1 clove garlic, minced</li><li>Salt and pepper to taste</li><li>Juice of 1/2 lemon</li></ul>	<ul><li>Heat olive oil in a skillet over medium heat.</li><li>Add garlic and mushrooms, sauté until mushrooms are tender.</li><li>Add spinach and cook until wilted.</li><li>Combine with cooked quinoa, season with salt, pepper, and lemon juice.</li><li>Serve warm.</li></ul>

SWEET POTATO AND BLACK BEAN TACOS

Ingredients:	Directions:
<ul><li>1 cup diced sweet potatoes</li><li>1 cup black beans, cooked</li><li>1 tablespoon olive oil</li><li>1/2 teaspoon cumin</li><li>1/2 teaspoon paprika</li><li>4 corn tortillas</li><li>Avocado slices, salsa, and lime wedges for serving</li></ul>	<ul><li>Toss sweet potatoes with olive oil, cumin, and paprika. Roast at 375°F for 20 minutes.</li><li>Warm black beans in a saucepan.</li><li>Assemble tacos with roasted sweet potatoes, black beans, avocado slices, and salsa on corn tortillas.</li><li>Serve with lime wedges.</li></ul>

TURMERIC LENTIL STEW

Ingredients:	Directions:
<ul><li>1 cup lentils</li><li>1 teaspoon turmeric powder</li><li>2 carrots, diced</li><li>1 onion, chopped</li><li>1 can diced tomatoes</li><li>4 cups vegetable broth</li><li>Salt and pepper to taste</li></ul>	<ul><li>Sauté onions and garlic in a pot until softened.</li><li>Add carrots, tomatoes, lentils, turmeric, and vegetable broth.</li><li>Simmer until lentils are tender, about 30 minutes.</li><li>Season with salt and pepper to taste.</li><li>Serve warm.</li></ul>

GREEK SALAD WITH PUMPKIN SEEDS

Ingredients:	Directions:
<ul><li>1 cup chopped cucumber</li><li>1 cup cherry tomatoes, halved</li><li>1/2 cup sliced red onion</li><li>1/2 cup Kalamata olives</li></ul>	<ul><li>In a large bowl, combine cucumber, cherry tomatoes, red onion, olives, feta cheese, and pumpkin seeds.</li><li>Drizzle with olive oil and lemon juice.</li></ul>

• 1/4 cup feta cheese, crumbled • 1/4 cup pumpkin seeds • 2 tablespoons olive oil • Juice of 1 lemon • Salt and pepper to taste	• Season with salt and pepper, then toss to combine. • Serve fresh.

ANTI-PARASITIC VEGETABLE CURRY WITH BROWN RICE

Ingredients:	Directions:
• 1 tablespoon coconut oil • 1 onion, chopped • 2 cloves garlic, minced • 1 tablespoon grated ginger • 1 tablespoon curry powder • 2 cups mixed vegetables (zucchini, bell peppers, carrots) • 1 can coconut milk • 1/2 cup vegetable broth • Salt and pepper to taste • 1 cup brown rice, cooked	• Heat coconut oil in a large pan over medium heat. • Add onion, garlic, and ginger, sauté until fragrant. • Stir in curry powder and mixed vegetables, cook for 5 minutes. • Add coconut milk and vegetable broth, simmer for 15 minutes. • Season with salt and pepper. • Serve over cooked brown rice.

ROASTED VEGETABLE AND LENTIL BOWL

Ingredients:	Directions:
• 1 cup cooked lentils • 1 cup roasted vegetables (carrots, sweet potatoes, Brussels sprouts) • 1 tablespoon olive oil • 1 tablespoon balsamic vinegar • 1/4 cup chopped fresh parsley • Salt and pepper to taste	• Combine cooked lentils and roasted vegetables in a bowl. • Drizzle with olive oil and balsamic vinegar. • Season with salt, pepper, and top with fresh parsley. • Serve warm.

QUINOA AND ROASTED VEGGIE BOWL

Ingredients:	Directions:
• 1 cup cooked quinoa • 1 cup roasted vegetables (broccoli, bell peppers, zucchini) • 1/4 cup hummus	• In a bowl, combine cooked quinoa and roasted vegetables. • Drizzle with olive oil and lemon juice. • Add a dollop of hummus on the side.

• 1 tablespoon olive oil • Juice of 1/2 lemon • Salt and pepper to taste	• Season with salt and pepper, and serve.

GREEK SALAD WITH FETA AND PUMPKIN SEEDS

Ingredients:	Directions:
• 1 cup chopped cucumber • 1 cup cherry tomatoes, halved • 1/2 cup sliced red onion • 1/2 cup Kalamata olives • 1/4 cup feta cheese, crumbled • 1/4 cup pumpkin seeds • 2 tablespoons olive oil • Juice of 1 lemon • Salt and pepper to taste	• Combine cucumber, cherry tomatoes, red onion, olives, feta cheese, and pumpkin seeds in a large bowl. • Drizzle with olive oil and lemon juice. • Season with salt and pepper, then toss to mix. • Serve fresh.

SEED PUMPKIN PESTO RECIPE

Ingredients:	Directions:
• 1 cup raw pumpkin seeds • 2 cups fresh basil leaves • 2 cloves garlic • 1/4 cup olive oil • 1/4 cup grated Parmesan cheese (optional) • Juice of 1 lemon • Salt and pepper to taste	• In a food processor, combine pumpkin seeds, basil leaves, and garlic. Pulse until the mixture is coarsely chopped. • With the food processor running, slowly drizzle in the olive oil until the mixture becomes smooth and creamy. • Add the Parmesan cheese (if using), lemon juice, salt, and pepper. Pulse a few more times to blend all ingredients. • Taste and adjust seasoning as needed. • Store in an airtight container in the refrigerator for up to one week.

DINNER RECIPES FOR THE PARASITE CLEANSE

GARLIC AND GINGER SOUP

Ingredients:

- 4 cloves garlic, minced
- 1-inch piece fresh ginger, minced
- 4 cups vegetable broth
- 2 carrots, sliced
- 2 celery stalks, sliced
- 1 tablespoon olive oil
- Salt and pepper to taste

Directions:

- Heat olive oil in a large pot over medium heat.
- Add garlic and ginger, sauté for 2-3 minutes until fragrant.
- Add carrots and celery, cook for another 5 minutes.
- Pour in the vegetable broth and bring to a boil.
- Reduce heat and simmer for 20 minutes until vegetables are tender.
- Season with salt and pepper to taste.
- Serve hot.

BAKED SALMON WITH STEAMED VEGETABLES

Ingredients:

- 2 salmon fillets
- 1 tablespoon olive oil
- Juice of 1 lemon
- 2 cloves garlic, minced
- 1 tablespoon fresh dill, chopped
- Salt and pepper to taste
- 2 cups mixed vegetables (broccoli, carrots, and zucchini)

Directions:

- Preheat the oven to 375°F (190°C).
- Place salmon fillets on a baking sheet lined with parchment paper.
- Drizzle olive oil, lemon juice over salmon, and sprinkle with garlic, dill, salt, and pepper.
- Bake for 20 minutes or until the salmon is cooked through.
- While salmon is baking, steam mixed vegetables until tender.
- Serve the baked salmon alongside steamed vegetables.

LENTIL AND VEGETABLE SOUP

Ingredients:

- 1 cup lentils
- 2 carrots, diced
- 2 celery stalks, diced
- 1 onion, chopped
- 4 cups vegetable broth
- 1 can diced tomatoes
- 1 tablespoon olive oil
- 2 cloves garlic, minced
- 1 teaspoon cumin

Directions:

- Heat olive oil in a large pot over medium heat.
- Add onion and garlic, sauté until softened.
- Add carrots, celery, cumin, and sauté for another 5 minutes.
- Stir in lentils, diced tomatoes, and vegetable broth.

	• Bring to a boil, then reduce heat and simmer for 30 minutes until lentils are tender.
• Salt and pepper to taste	• Season with salt and pepper to taste.
	• Serve hot.

STUFFED BELL PEPPERS

Ingredients:	Directions:
• 4 bell peppers, halved and seeds removed • 1 cup cooked quinoa • 1/2 cup black beans, drained and rinsed • 1/2 cup corn kernels • 1/2 cup diced tomatoes • 1/4 cup chopped cilantro • 1 teaspoon cumin • 1 tablespoon olive oil • Salt and pepper to taste	• Preheat the oven to 375°F (190°C). • In a bowl, mix cooked quinoa, black beans, corn, diced tomatoes, cilantro, cumin, olive oil, salt, and pepper. • Fill each bell pepper half with the quinoa mixture. • Place stuffed peppers in a baking dish and bake for 25-30 minutes until peppers are tender. • Serve hot.

GINGER AND TURMERIC ROASTED VEGETABLES

Ingredients:	Directions:
• 4 cups mixed vegetables (sweet potatoes, carrots, cauliflower) • 1 teaspoon turmeric powder • 1-inch piece fresh ginger, grated • 2 tablespoons olive oil • Salt and pepper to taste	• Preheat the oven to 400°F (200°C). • In a large bowl, toss vegetables with turmeric, grated ginger, olive oil, salt, and pepper. • Spread the vegetables evenly on a baking sheet. • Roast for 20-25 minutes, stirring halfway through, until vegetables are tender and golden. • Serve warm.

HERB-CRUSTED BAKED FISH

Ingredients:	Directions:
• 2 white fish fillets (such as cod or tilapia) • 1/4 cup breadcrumbs • 1 tablespoon fresh parsley, chopped • 1 tablespoon fresh thyme, chopped	• Preheat the oven to 375°F (190°C). • Mix breadcrumbs, parsley, thyme, olive oil, salt, and pepper in a small bowl. • Press the breadcrumb mixture onto the fish fillets to form a crust.

• 1 tablespoon olive oil • Salt and pepper to taste • Lemon wedges for serving	• Place fish fillets on a baking sheet lined with parchment paper. • Bake for 15-20 minutes until the fish is cooked through and the crust is golden. • Serve with lemon wedges.

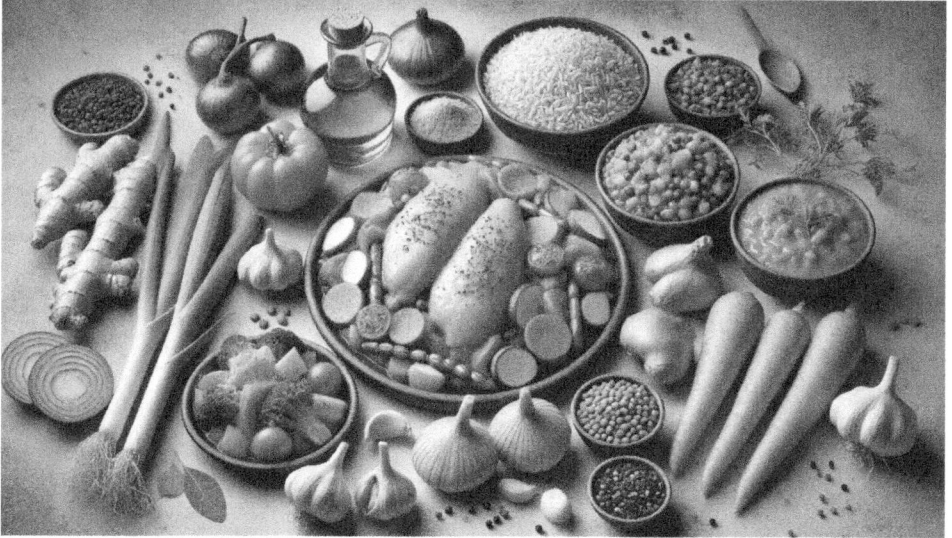

TURMERIC AND GINGER CHICKEN

Ingredients:	Directions:
• 2 chicken breasts • 1 teaspoon turmeric powder • 1-inch piece fresh ginger, grated • 2 cloves garlic, minced • 2 tablespoons olive oil • Salt and pepper to taste	• In a bowl, mix turmeric, ginger, garlic, olive oil, salt, and pepper. • Marinate chicken breasts in the mixture for at least 30 minutes. • Preheat the oven to 375°F (190°C). • Place chicken breasts on a baking sheet and bake for 25-30 minutes until cooked through. • Serve hot with a side of steamed vegetables.

ZUCCHINI NOODLES WITH PESTO

Ingredients:	Directions:
• 2 zucchinis, spiralized into noodles • 1/2 cup homemade or store-bought pesto • 1 tablespoon olive oil • 1/4 cup cherry tomatoes, halved • 1/4 cup grated Parmesan cheese (optional) • Salt and pepper to taste	• Heat olive oil in a skillet over medium heat. • Add zucchini noodles and sauté for 2-3 minutes until just tender. • Stir in pesto and cherry tomatoes, cooking for another 2 minutes. • Season with salt and pepper. • Top with grated Parmesan cheese, if desired, and serve.

COCONUT OIL STIR-FRY

Ingredients:	Directions:
• 2 cups mixed vegetables (broccoli, bell peppers, carrots) • 2 tablespoons coconut oil • 2 cloves garlic, minced • 2 tablespoons soy sauce • 1 tablespoon fresh ginger, grated • 1/2 cup cooked brown rice	• Heat coconut oil in a large skillet or wok over medium-high heat. • Add garlic and ginger, sauté for 1 minute. • Add mixed vegetables and stir-fry until tender-crisp, about 5-7 minutes. • Stir in soy sauce and cook for another 2 minutes. • Serve over cooked brown rice.

TURMERIC AND GINGER CHICKEN STIR-FRY

Ingredients:	Directions:
• 2 chicken breasts, sliced • 1 teaspoon turmeric powder • 1-inch piece fresh ginger, grated • 2 cloves garlic, minced • 2 cups mixed vegetables (bell peppers, snap peas, carrots) • 2 tablespoons olive oil • 2 tablespoons soy sauce • Salt and pepper to taste	• In a bowl, mix chicken slices with turmeric, ginger, garlic, and a pinch of salt. • Heat olive oil in a skillet over medium-high heat. • Add chicken and cook until browned and cooked through. • Add mixed vegetables and stir-fry for 5-7 minutes. • Stir in soy sauce, cooking for another 2 minutes. • Serve hot.

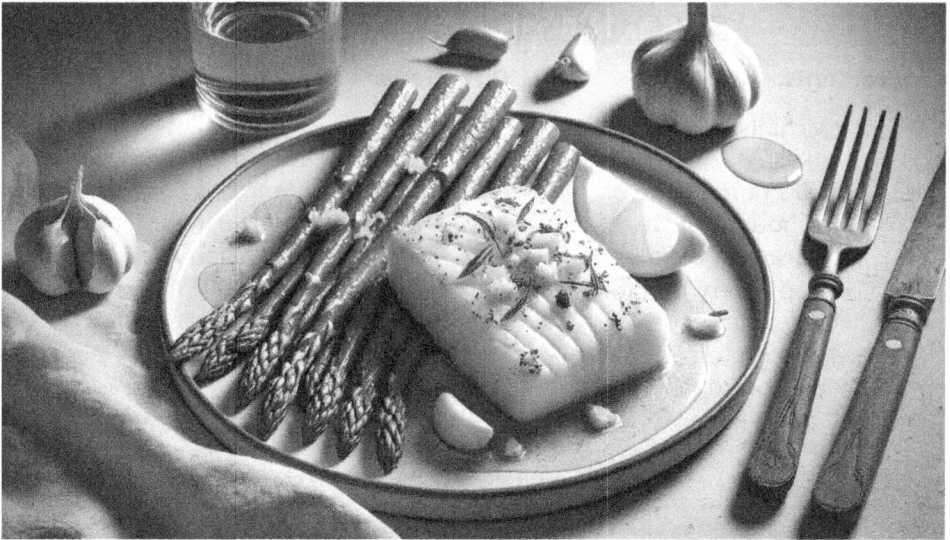

BAKED COD WITH ASPARAGUS

Ingredients:

- 2 cod fillets
- 1 tablespoon olive oil
- Juice of 1 lemon
- 2 cloves garlic, minced
- 1 bunch asparagus, trimmed
- Salt and pepper to taste

Directions:

- Preheat the oven to 375°F (190°C).
- Place cod fillets and asparagus on a baking sheet lined with parchment paper.
- Drizzle with olive oil and lemon juice, then sprinkle with garlic, salt, and pepper.
- Bake for 20 minutes or until the fish is cooked through and asparagus is tender.
- Serve hot.

STUFFED ZUCCHINI BOATS

Ingredients:

- 2 zucchinis, halved lengthwise and seeds removed
- 1 cup cooked quinoa
- 1/2 cup diced tomatoes
- 1/4 cup diced bell peppers
- 1/4 cup grated Parmesan cheese (optional)
- 1 tablespoon olive oil
- Salt and pepper to taste

Directions:

- Preheat the oven to 375°F (190°C).
- In a bowl, mix cooked quinoa, diced tomatoes, bell peppers, olive oil, salt, and pepper.
- Fill zucchini halves with the quinoa mixture.
- Place zucchini boats on a baking sheet and sprinkle with Parmesan cheese, if using.
- Bake for 20 minutes until zucchini is tender and filling is heated through.

	• Serve hot.

HERB-ROASTED CHICKEN WITH STEAMED GREENS

Ingredients:	Directions:
• 2 chicken breasts • 1 tablespoon olive oil • 1 tablespoon fresh rosemary, chopped • 1 tablespoon fresh thyme, chopped • Salt and pepper to taste • 2 cups mixed greens (kale, spinach, Swiss chard)	• Preheat the oven to 375°F (190°C). • Rub chicken breasts with olive oil, rosemary, thyme, salt, and pepper. • Place on a baking sheet and roast for 25-30 minutes until cooked through. • While the chicken is roasting, steam mixed greens until tender. • Serve the roasted chicken with a side of steamed greens.

HERB-ROASTED CHICKEN WITH STEAMED BROCCOLI

Ingredients:	Directions:
• 2 chicken breasts • 1 tablespoon olive oil • 1 tablespoon fresh parsley, chopped • 1 tablespoon fresh dill, chopped • Salt and pepper to taste • 2 cups broccoli florets	• Preheat the oven to 375°F (190°C). • Rub chicken breasts with olive oil, parsley, dill, salt, and pepper. • Place on a baking sheet and roast for 25-30 minutes until cooked through. • Steam broccoli florets until tender. • Serve the herb-roasted chicken with steamed broccoli.

Snack Recipes for the Parasite Cleanse

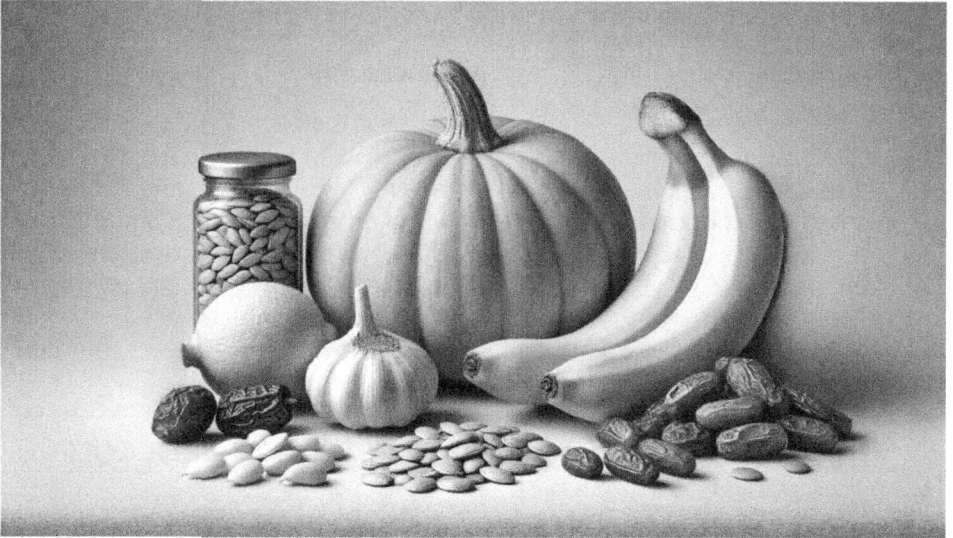

ROASTED PUMPKIN SEEDS

Ingredients:	Directions:
• 1 cup raw pumpkin seeds • 1 tablespoon olive oil • 1/2 teaspoon sea salt • 1/4 teaspoon paprika (optional)	• Preheat the oven to 350°F (175°C). • In a bowl, toss pumpkin seeds with olive oil, sea salt, and paprika (if using). • Spread the seeds evenly on a baking sheet. • Roast for 15-20 minutes, stirring occasionally, until golden brown and crispy. • Let cool and store in an airtight container.

FRESH FRUIT WITH ALMOND BUTTER

Ingredients:	Directions:
• 1 apple or banana, sliced • 2 tablespoons almond butter	• Slice the apple or banana into thin pieces. • Arrange the fruit slices on a plate. • Serve with almond butter for dipping.

COCONUT OIL ENERGY BALLS

Ingredients:	Directions:
• 1 cup rolled oats • 1/2 cup shredded coconut • 1/4 cup coconut oil, melted • 1/4 cup honey • 1/4 cup dried fruits (such as cranberries or raisins) • 1/4 cup chopped nuts (optional)	• In a bowl, mix oats, shredded coconut, dried fruits, and nuts (if using). • Add melted coconut oil and honey, stirring until well combined. • Form the mixture into small balls using your hands. • Place the energy balls on a baking sheet and refrigerate for 30 minutes until firm. • Store in an airtight container in the refrigerator.

FRESH VEGGIES WITH PUMPKIN SEED PESTO

Ingredients:	Directions:
• 1 cup assorted fresh veggies (carrot sticks, cucumber slices, bell pepper strips) • 1/2 cup pumpkin seed pesto (see recipe in lunch options)	• Arrange the fresh veggies on a platter. • Serve with pumpkin seed pesto for dipping.

PUMPKIN SEED ENERGY BITES

Ingredients:	Directions:
• 1/2 cup pumpkin seeds • 1/2 cup dates, pitted • 1/4 cup almond butter • 1 tablespoon chia seeds • 1/4 teaspoon sea salt	• In a food processor, blend pumpkin seeds and dates until finely chopped. • Add almond butter, chia seeds, and sea salt, processing until the mixture comes together. • Roll the mixture into small balls using your hands. • Refrigerate for 30 minutes until firm. • Store in an airtight container in the refrigerator.

FRESH PINEAPPLE CHUNKS

Ingredients:	Directions:
• 1 fresh pineapple, peeled and cut into chunks	• Peel and core the pineapple, then cut it into bite-sized chunks. • Serve immediately or store in an airtight container in the refrigerator.

HERBAL LEMONADE WITH FRESH MINT

Ingredients:	Directions:
• 1 lemon, juiced • 1 tablespoon honey • 2 cups water • A handful of fresh mint leaves	• In a pitcher, combine lemon juice, honey, and water. Stir until the honey is dissolved. • Add fresh mint leaves and stir. • Serve chilled over ice.

RAW VEGGIE STICKS WITH HUMMUS

Ingredients:	Directions:
• 1 cup assorted raw veggies (carrot sticks, cucumber slices, celery sticks) • 1/2 cup hummus	• Arrange raw veggie sticks on a platter. • Serve with hummus for dipping.

SLICED APPLES WITH CINNAMON

Ingredients:	Directions:
• 1 apple, sliced • 1/4 teaspoon ground cinnamon	• Slice the apple into thin pieces. • Arrange the apple slices on a plate. • Sprinkle ground cinnamon over the apple slices. • Serve immediately.

FRESH PINEAPPLE WITH MINT

Ingredients:	Directions:
• 1 cup fresh pineapple chunks • A handful of fresh mint leaves, chopped	• Arrange fresh pineapple chunks on a plate. • Sprinkle with chopped mint leaves. • Serve chilled.

PUMPKIN SEED PESTO ON CRACKERS

Ingredients:	Directions:
• 1/2 cup pumpkin seed pesto (see recipe in lunch options) • 1 cup whole-grain crackers	• Spread pumpkin seed pesto on whole-grain crackers. • Arrange on a serving platter. • Serve as a light snack.

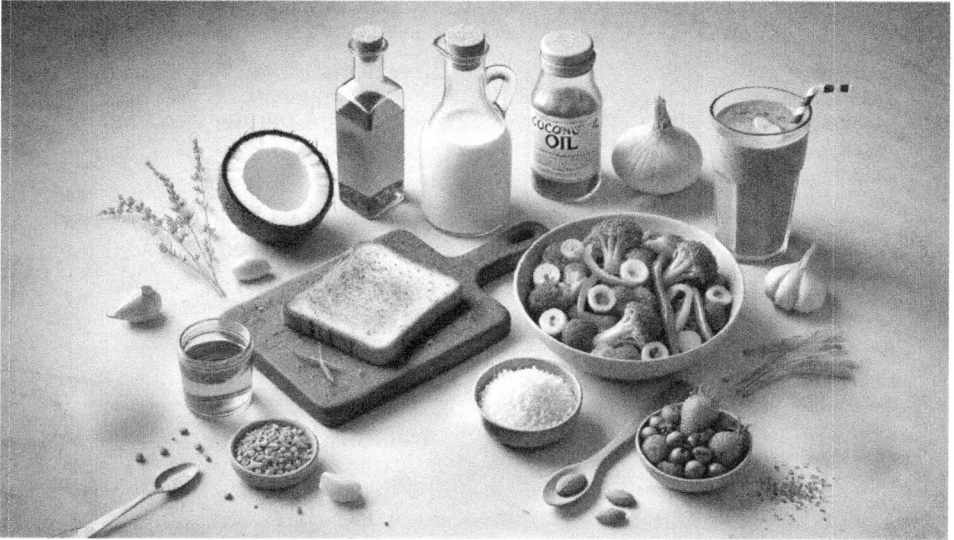

MIXED NUTS AND SEEDS

Ingredients:	Directions:
• 1/2 cup mixed nuts (almonds, walnuts, cashews) • 1/2 cup mixed seeds (pumpkin seeds, sunflower seeds)	• Combine mixed nuts and seeds in a bowl. • Serve as a quick and nutritious snack.

FRESH FRUIT SALAD WITH COCONUT FLAKES

Ingredients:	Directions:
• 1 cup mixed fresh fruit (such as berries, melon, kiwi) • 2 tablespoons unsweetened coconut flakes	• Chop the fresh fruit into bite-sized pieces. • Toss fruit in a bowl and sprinkle with coconut flakes. • Serve immediately.

NUT BUTTER ON APPLE SLICES

Ingredients:	Directions:
• 1 apple, sliced • 2 tablespoons nut butter (almond, peanut, or cashew)	• Slice the apple into thin pieces. • Spread nut butter on each slice. • Arrange on a plate and serve.

COCONUT OIL AND BERRY SMOOTHIE BOWL

Ingredients:	Directions:
• 1 cup mixed berries • 1 banana • 1 tablespoon coconut oil • 1/2 cup Greek yogurt • 1/2 cup almond milk • Toppings: fresh fruit, nuts, seeds	• Blend mixed berries, banana, coconut oil, Greek yogurt, and almond milk until smooth. • Pour into a bowl and top with fresh fruit, nuts, and seeds. • Serve immediately.

PUMPKIN SEED AND DATE BALLS

Ingredients:	Directions:
• 1 cup pumpkin seeds • 1/2 cup dates, pitted • 1 tablespoon honey • 1/4 teaspoon sea salt	• In a food processor, blend pumpkin seeds and dates until finely chopped. • Add honey and sea salt, processing until the mixture comes together. • Roll the mixture into small balls using your hands. • Refrigerate for 30 minutes until firm. • Store in an airtight container in the refrigerator.

GINGER AND TURMERIC INFUSION

Ingredients:	Directions:
• 1-inch piece fresh ginger, sliced • 1-inch piece fresh turmeric root, sliced • 1 teaspoon honey (optional) • 2 cups water	• Bring 2 cups of water to a boil in a small saucepan. • Add the sliced ginger and turmeric root to the boiling water. • Reduce heat and simmer for 10 minutes. • Strain the infusion into a cup. • Add honey if desired for sweetness. Stir well and enjoy warm.

WORMWOOD TEA

Ingredients:	Directions:
• 1 teaspoon dried wormwood leaves • 1 cup boiling water	• Place the dried wormwood leaves in a tea infuser or teapot. • Pour boiling water over the leaves and cover. • Let steep for 10 minutes to allow the beneficial compounds to infuse into the water. • Strain the tea into a cup and discard the leaves. • Drink while warm. Note: Due to its bitter taste, you may add a small amount of honey or lemon if needed.

CLOVE AND CINNAMON TEA

Ingredients:	Directions:
• 4 whole cloves • 1 cinnamon stick • 2 cups water	• Bring 2 cups of water to a boil in a saucepan. • Add the cloves and cinnamon stick to the boiling water. • Reduce the heat and simmer for 10 minutes to extract the flavors and beneficial oils. • Strain the tea into a cup. • Enjoy warm, optionally sweetened with honey or a slice of lemon.

BLACK WALNUT HULL TEA

Ingredients:	Directions:
• 1 teaspoon dried black walnut hull • 1 cup boiling water	• Place the dried black walnut hull in a tea infuser or directly in a cup. • Pour boiling water over the walnut hull and cover the cup. • Allow it to steep for 10 minutes. • Strain the tea if necessary. • Drink warm. Due to its strong flavor, you may add a bit of honey or lemon juice for taste.

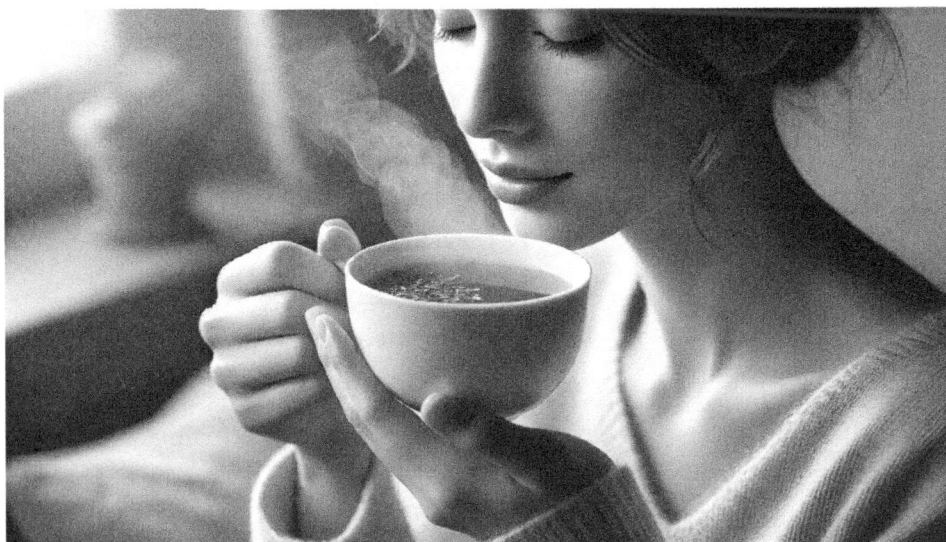

HOLY BASIL (TULSI) TEA

Ingredients:	Directions:
• 1 teaspoon dried holy basil (tulsi) leaves • 1 cup boiling water	• Add the dried holy basil leaves to a tea infuser or teapot. • Pour 1 cup of boiling water over the leaves. • Cover and let steep for 5-10 minutes to release the aromatic oils and beneficial compounds. • Strain the tea into a cup and discard the leaves. • Enjoy the tea warm, with optional honey or lemon for added flavor.

GINGER AND APPLE JUICE

Ingredients:	Directions:
• 1-inch piece fresh ginger • 2 green apples • Juice of 1 lemon	• Peel and slice the fresh ginger. • Core and chop the green apples into smaller pieces suitable for your juicer. • Juice the ginger and apples together in a juicer. • Add the juice of 1 lemon to the mixture for an extra detoxifying boost. • Stir well and drink immediately to benefit from the fresh enzymes and nutrients.

FENNEL AND THYME TEA

Ingredients:	Directions:
• 1 teaspoon fennel seeds • 1 teaspoon dried thyme leaves • 1 cup boiling water • Honey or lemon (optional)	• Place the fennel seeds and dried thyme leaves in a tea infuser or teapot. • Pour 1 cup of boiling water over the fennel and thyme. • Cover and let steep for 10 minutes to allow the herbs to release their essential oils and beneficial compounds. • Strain the tea into a cup and discard the seeds and leaves. • Enjoy the tea warm. You can add honey or a slice of lemon for additional flavor if desired.

PARASITE CLEANSE PROGRAM

Welcome to the Parasite Cleanse Program, a journey towards a healthier, more vibrant you. This chapter provides a comprehensive, 30-day plan to cleanse your body and restore balance, focusing on anti-parasitic foods, herbs, and natural practices. The goal is to support your body's natural ability to eliminate parasites while nourishing it with nutrient-dense meals.

As you begin, remember that this program is flexible. Each phase is designed to guide you through a gentle yet effective process, starting with preparation and moving through intensive and deep cleansing, before finally restoring your body to its optimal state. If a recipe doesn't quite suit your tastes or needs, feel free to make adjustments. The key is to listen to your body and make this cleanse your own.

Throughout this program, consistency and self-awareness are your best allies. Be patient with yourself and trust that each step you take is bringing you closer to your health goals. Regular maintenance, including weekly, monthly, and seasonal detox practices, will help keep your body in balance long after the cleanse is over.

Embrace this opportunity to connect more deeply with your body and its needs. This is more than just a cleanse—it's a step towards a healthier, more mindful way of living. Enjoy the process, stay committed, and watch as your health transforms.

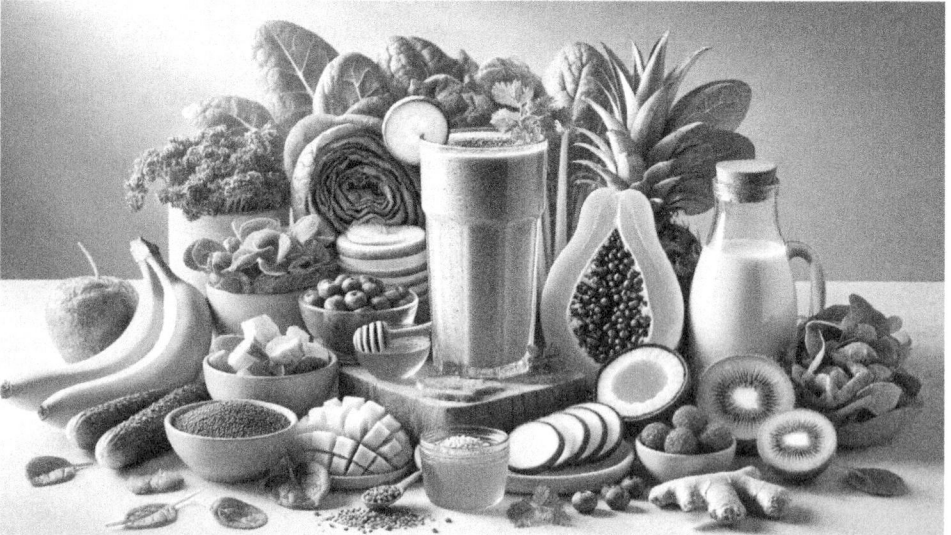

30-Day Program: Step by Step

Week 1: Preparation Phase

Focus: Hydration, gentle detoxification, and dietary adjustments.

Days 1-3: Hydration and Diet Adjustment: During these first few days, focus on increasing your water intake and making dietary adjustments to prepare your body for the cleanse. Your meals should be light, nutrient-rich, and designed to hydrate and support your body's natural detox processes.

Breakfast Options:

- o Green Detox Smoothie
- o Cilantro and Pineapple Juice

Lunch Options:

- o Quinoa and Avocado Salad
- o Chickpea Salad Wrap

Dinner Options:

- o Garlic and Ginger Soup
- o Baked Salmon with Steamed Vegetables

Snacks:

- o Roasted Pumpkin Seeds
- o Fresh Fruit with Almond Butter

Teas & Infusions:

- o Ginger and Turmeric Infusion
- o Wormwood Tea

Days 4-7: Gentle Detox: As your body adjusts, introduce gentle detox practices and continue with balanced meals. The aim is to maintain variety and include foods that gently support detoxification.

Breakfast Options:

- Papaya Seed Smoothie
- Overnight Oats with Pumpkin Seeds and Cinnamon
- Cilantro and Pineapple Juice
- Chia Seed Pudding with Fresh Berries

Lunch Options:

- Vegetable Stir-Fry with Tofu
- Roasted Pumpkin Seeds and Mixed Green Salad
- Fermented Vegetable Salad
- Pumpkin Seed Pesto Salad

Dinner Options:

- Lentil and Vegetable Soup
- Stuffed Bell Peppers
- Ginger and Turmeric Roasted Vegetables
- Herb-Crusted Baked Fish

Snacks:

- Coconut Oil Energy Balls
- Fresh Veggies with Pumpkin Seed Pesto

Teas & Infusions:

- Clove and Cinnamon Tea
- Black Walnut Hull Tea

Week 2: Intensive Cleansing Phase

Focus: Anti-parasitic foods and herbs to target parasites more aggressively.

Days 8-10: Intensive Cleanse: Ramp up with targeted anti-parasitic foods and supplements. Meals should focus on ingredients known for their cleansing properties.

Breakfast Options:

- o Papaya Seed Smoothie
- o Anti-Parasitic Grain Bowl
- o Coconut Oil and Berry Smoothie
- o Scrambled Eggs with Turmeric and Spinach

Lunch Options:

- o Pumpkin Seed Pesto Pasta
- o Spinach and Mushroom Quinoa Bowl
- o Sweet Potato and Black Bean Tacos
- o Turmeric Lentil Stew

Dinner Options:

- o Turmeric and Ginger Chicken
- o Zucchini Noodles with Pesto
- o Coconut Oil Stir-Fry
- o Baked Cod with Asparagus

Snacks:

- o Pumpkin Seed Energy Bites
- o Fresh Pineapple Chunks

Teas & Infusions:

- o Holy Basil (Tulsi) Tea
- o Ginger and Apple Juice

Days 11-14: Continued Intensive Cleanse: Maintain intensity with potent anti-parasitic ingredients while keeping your meals varied and nutritious.

Breakfast Options:

- o Coconut Oil and Berry Smoothie
- o Ginger and Apple Juice
- o Anti-Parasitic Chia Pudding with Coconut Milk
- o Spinach and Avocado Toast

Lunch Options:

- o Turmeric Lentil Stew
- o Greek Salad with Pumpkin Seeds
- o Anti-Parasitic Vegetable Curry with Brown Rice
- o Roasted Vegetable and Lentil Bowl

Dinner Options:

- o Coconut Oil Stir-Fry
- o Baked Cod with Asparagus
- o Anti-Parasitic Vegetable Curry with Brown Rice
- o Roasted Vegetable and Lentil Bowl

Snacks:

- o Herbal Lemonade with Fresh Mint
- o Raw Veggie Sticks with Hummus

Teas & Infusions:

- o Clove and Cinnamon Tea
- o Ginger and Turmeric Infusion

Week 3: Deep Cleansing Phase

Focus: Potent anti-parasitic foods, deep detoxification, and support for the body.

Days 15-17: Deep Cleanse: Continue to cleanse with powerful anti-parasitic foods while providing your body with necessary nutrients to support detoxification.

Breakfast Options:

- Ginger and Apple Juice
- Anti-Parasitic Chia Pudding with Coconut Milk
- Green Detox Smoothie
- Papaya Seed Smoothie

Lunch Options:

- Turmeric Lentil Stew
- Quinoa and Roasted Veggie Bowl
- Greek Salad with Pumpkin Seeds
- Lentil and Vegetable Soup

Dinner Options:

- Ginger and Turmeric Roasted Vegetables
- Herb-Crusted Baked Fish
- Turmeric and Ginger Chicken Stir-Fry
- Stuffed Zucchini Boats

Snacks:

- Coconut Oil Energy Balls
- Sliced Apples with Cinnamon

Teas & Infusions:

- Black Walnut Hull Tea
- Wormwood Tea

Days 18-21: Deep Cleanse Intensified: Maintain a robust cleansing regimen with a variety of meals that continue to target parasites effectively.

Breakfast Options:

- Coconut Oil and Berry Smoothie Bowl
- Green Detox Smoothie
- Cilantro and Pineapple Juice
- Coconut Oil Energy Balls

Lunch Options:

- Anti-Parasitic Vegetable Curry with Brown Rice
- Greek Salad with Feta and Pumpkin Seeds
- Pumpkin Seed Pesto Pasta
- Spinach and Mushroom Quinoa Bowl

Dinner Options:

- Baked Herb-Crusted Fish with Steamed Greens
- Turmeric and Ginger Chicken Stir-Fry
- Zucchini Noodles with Pesto
- Herb-Roasted Chicken with Steamed

Snacks:

- Fresh Pineapple with Mint
- Pumpkin Seed and Date Balls

Teas & Infusions:

- Holy Basil (Tulsi) Tea
- Ginger and Turmeric Infusion

Week 4: Restoration Phase

Focus: Restoring balance, rebuilding strength, and supporting long-term health.

Days 22-24: Begin Restoration: Shift your focus to restoring and balancing the body, with meals designed to replenish nutrients and support healing.

Breakfast Options:

- Coconut Oil and Berry Smoothie
- Green Detox Smoothie with Spirulina
- Papaya Seed Smoothie
- Anti-Parasitic Overnight Oats with Pumpkin Seeds

Lunch Options:

- Lentil and Vegetable Soup
- Greek Salad with Pumpkin Seeds
- Roasted Vegetable and Lentil Bowl
- Quinoa and Avocado Salad

Dinner Options:

- Ginger and Turmeric Roasted Vegetables
- Stuffed Zucchini Boats
- Coconut Oil Stir-Fry with Mixed Vegetables
- Herb-Roasted Chicken with Steamed Broccoli

Snacks:

- Pumpkin Seed Pesto on Crackers
- Mixed Nuts and Seeds

Teas & Infusions:

- Ginger and Turmeric Infusion
- Clove and Cinnamon Tea

Days 25-30: Full Restoration and Maintenance: Complete the cleanse by fully restoring your body's strength and resilience. Emphasize nutrient-dense meals and gentle detox practices.

Breakfast Options:

- o Papaya Seed Smoothie
- o Anti-Parasitic Overnight Oats with Pumpkin Seeds
- o Cilantro and Pineapple Juice
- o Green Detox Smoothie

Lunch Options:

- o Quinoa and Avocado Salad
- o Roasted Vegetable and Lentil Bowl
- o Turmeric Lentil Stew
- o Lentil and Vegetable Soup

Dinner Options:

- o Coconut Oil Stir-Fry with Mixed Vegetables
- o Herb-Roasted Chicken with Steamed Broccoli
- o Baked Salmon with Steamed Vegetables
- o Stuffed Zucchini Boats

Snacks:

- o Fresh Fruit Salad with Coconut Flakes
- o Nut Butter on Apple Slices

Teas & Infusions:

- o Wormwood Tea
- o Holy Basil (Tulsi) Tea

This detailed 30-day parasite cleanse plan provides a diverse range of anti-parasitic recipes and herbal infusions to ensure a balanced and effective cleanse. By rotating different meals and beverages, the program maintains interest and engagement while delivering maximum health benefits.

Maintenance Program

Congratulations on completing the 30-day parasite cleanse! The journey to maintaining a parasite-free body doesn't end here. It's important to continue nurturing your body with regular detox practices and mindful eating habits to ensure long-term health and vitality. Here's how you can keep parasites at bay and support your body's natural defenses:

Weekly Detox Practices

To keep your body in top shape, integrate weekly detox practices into your routine. These small but powerful habits help flush out toxins and support your body's detoxification process.

Green Detox Smoothie: Once or twice a week, enjoy a refreshing Green Detox Smoothie. Blend together 1 cup of spinach, 1 cup of kale, 1 green apple, 1/2 cucumber, the juice of 1/2 a lemon, 1 tablespoon of chia seeds, and 1 cup of water. This nutrient-packed smoothie helps cleanse your system and boost your energy levels.

Turmeric and Ginger Tea: A couple of times a week, sip on this warming tea. Boil 1 inch each of ginger and turmeric root in 2 cups of water, simmer for 15 minutes, strain, and enjoy. This tea not only aids digestion but also has anti-inflammatory properties, making it a great choice for ongoing health maintenance.

Monthly Maintenance Cleanse

Set aside one day each month for a mini-cleanse to reset your system and reinforce your body's defenses against parasites. This day should focus on simple, nourishing meals that promote detoxification.

Breakfast: Start your day with **Wormwood Tea**. Steep 1 teaspoon of dried wormwood leaves in 1 cup of boiling water for 5-10 minutes. Strain and drink. This tea is known for its antiparasitic properties and is an excellent way to kick off your cleanse day.

Lunch: For lunch, have a **Pumpkin Seed Pesto**. Blend 1 cup of fresh basil leaves, 1/2 cup of pumpkin seeds, 2 cloves of garlic, 1/4 cup of olive oil, and 1/4 cup of grated Parmesan cheese (optional). Season with salt and pepper to taste. This nutrient-rich pesto is packed with antiparasitic ingredients and makes a delicious, healthy meal.

Dinner: End your day with a comforting bowl of **Turmeric Lentil Stew**. Sauté 1 chopped onion and 2 cloves of minced garlic, then add 1 cup of lentils, 4 cups of vegetable broth, 1 tablespoon of turmeric powder, 1 teaspoon of cumin, and 1 cup of spinach. Simmer for 30 minutes. This stew not only warms the soul but also helps cleanse the body from within.

Seasonal Cleansing Strategies

Every three months, commit to a seasonal cleanse to rejuvenate your body and bolster your defenses against parasites. Each cleanse is tailored to the season, taking advantage of seasonal ingredients and addressing specific health needs.

Spring Cleanse: Spring is the perfect time to rejuvenate and refresh your body. Start with a **Papaya Seed Smoothie** for breakfast, then enjoy a light **Quinoa and Avocado Salad** for lunch. For dinner, try **Turmeric and Ginger Chicken**, a dish that combines anti-inflammatory and antiparasitic ingredients to cleanse and nourish.

Summer Cleanse: Keep cool and hydrated with a **Cilantro and Pineapple Juice** to start your day. For lunch, savor a bowl of **Garlic and Ginger Soup**, and finish with a **Coconut Oil Stir-Fry** for dinner. These meals are designed to refresh your system and keep you energized through the warm months.

Fall Cleanse: As the weather cools, warm up with a **Ginger and Apple Juice** for breakfast, followed by a hearty **Lentil and Vegetable Soup** for lunch. For a healthy snack, enjoy **Pumpkin Seed Energy Bites**. These meals are rich in nutrients and help prepare your body for the colder season.

Winter Cleanse: Combat the cold with a **Ginger and Turmeric Infusion** to start your day. Enjoy **Turmeric and Ginger Roasted Vegetables** for lunch and snack on **Coconut Oil Energy Balls** to keep your energy levels high. These meals are designed to nourish and strengthen your body during the winter months.

By following this maintenance program, you continue to protect your body from parasites and promote overall health and well-being. These practices, combined with delicious, nutrient-dense recipes, provide a holistic approach to maintaining a clean, balanced body.

Conclusion

Starting a parasite cleanse can greatly improve your well-being, and this 30-day program is here to guide you every step of the way. With a clear plan for preparation, cleansing, and restoration, you'll use natural foods and herbs to support your body's defenses.

Stay consistent, and feel free to adjust recipes to suit your tastes. Regular detox practices, both during and after the cleanse, will help maintain your results and promote long-term health. Trust the process, listen to your body, and be patient. This guide is here to help you achieve lasting, positive changes for your health.

7. Managing Side Effects

A parasite cleanse is a significant step towards better health, but it can come with challenges. Understanding and managing side effects, particularly die-off reactions (Herxheimer reaction), is crucial for a smooth experience. These reactions occur when parasites die rapidly, releasing toxins that can cause symptoms like headaches, fatigue, and nausea.

While uncomfortable, these symptoms indicate the cleanse is working. Managing them effectively, along with boosting your immune system, is key to a successful cleanse. Immune-boosting supplements and stress reduction techniques play vital roles in this process.

This section provides strategies to handle die-off reactions and support your immune system. By understanding these processes and adopting practical measures, you can navigate your cleanse with confidence, emerging healthier and more energized.

DIE-OFF REACTIONS AND HOW TO MANAGE THEM

When embarking on a parasite cleanse, one of the most challenging aspects can be dealing with die-off reactions. These reactions, also known as Herxheimer reactions, occur when the parasites in your body die off and release toxins into your system faster than your body can eliminate them. While these reactions are a sign that the cleanse is working, they can be uncomfortable and sometimes overwhelming. Understanding die-off reactions and knowing how to manage them is crucial for making your parasite cleanse a successful and bearable experience.

Understanding Die-Off Reactions

Die-off reactions happen when large numbers of parasites are killed off by the cleanse, releasing a significant amount of toxins into the bloodstream. This sudden influx of toxins can overwhelm the body's detoxification pathways, leading to a variety of symptoms. These reactions are not unique to parasite cleanses; they can occur during any type of detoxification process where there is a rapid die-off of harmful organisms in the body.

Common symptoms of die-off reactions include headaches, fatigue, muscle and joint pain, nausea, digestive issues, chills, fever, and brain fog. These symptoms can vary in intensity from person to person and can last from a few days to several weeks, depending on the severity of the infestation and the individual's overall health.

It's essential to recognize that die-off reactions, though uncomfortable, are a normal part of the cleansing process. They indicate that the cleanse is effective and that your body is working hard to eliminate the parasites and their toxins. However, understanding the mechanisms behind these reactions and knowing how to support your body through them can significantly reduce discomfort and make the cleanse more manageable.

Strategies to Mitigate Side Effects

Managing die-off reactions effectively involves supporting your body's detoxification processes, reducing inflammation, and ensuring adequate rest and hydration. Here are some strategies to help mitigate the side effects of die-off reactions:

Stay Hydrated: Drinking plenty of water is crucial during a cleanse. Water helps flush out toxins and supports kidney function. Aim to drink at least half your body weight in ounces of water daily. Adding a squeeze of lemon can provide additional detoxifying benefits.

Support Your Liver: The liver plays a central role in detoxification. Supporting liver function can help manage die-off reactions. Herbs like milk thistle, dandelion root, and burdock root are known for their liver-supporting properties. Including these herbs in your routine can aid the liver in processing and eliminating toxins.

Incorporate Detox Baths: Epsom salt baths can help draw out toxins through the skin and provide relief from muscle aches and pains. Adding a few drops of essential oils like lavender or eucalyptus can enhance the relaxing and detoxifying effects.

Boost Your Immune System: A strong immune system can help your body cope with the increased toxic load. Consuming immune-boosting foods such as garlic, ginger, turmeric, and foods rich in vitamin C and zinc can support your immune response.

Use Activated Charcoal: Activated charcoal can bind to toxins in the digestive tract and help remove them from the body. Taking activated charcoal supplements can reduce the overall toxic load and alleviate symptoms of die-off reactions. Ensure to take it away from meals and other supplements, as it can interfere with nutrient absorption.

Rest and Gentle Exercise: Rest is vital for allowing your body to heal and detoxify. Ensure you get plenty of sleep and listen to your body's need for rest. Gentle exercises like walking, yoga, or stretching can promote circulation and support the lymphatic system in removing toxins.

Maintain a Nutrient-Dense Diet: Eating a diet rich in nutrients supports your body's natural detoxification processes. Focus on consuming plenty of fresh vegetables, fruits, whole grains, and lean proteins. Avoid processed foods, refined sugars, and alcohol, as they can burden your detoxification pathways.

Monitor Your Symptoms: Keep track of your symptoms and their intensity. This can help you identify any patterns or triggers and adjust your cleanse protocol accordingly. If symptoms become severe or unmanageable, it's essential to consult with a healthcare professional for guidance.

Supportive Supplements: Certain supplements can help mitigate the effects of die-off reactions. Omega-3 fatty acids, found in fish oil and flaxseed oil, have anti-inflammatory properties. Probiotics can help maintain gut health and support the elimination of toxins. Antioxidants like vitamin E and selenium can protect your cells from oxidative damage caused by toxins.

Herbal Teas and Infusions: Drinking herbal teas can provide additional support during a cleanse. Teas made from herbs like peppermint, chamomile, and nettle can soothe the digestive system, reduce inflammation, and support detoxification. These teas are gentle on the body and can be consumed throughout the day.

Breathing Exercises and Meditation: Stress can exacerbate die-off symptoms. Incorporating breathing exercises and meditation into your daily routine can help reduce stress and support your body's healing process. Techniques such as deep breathing, progressive muscle relaxation, and mindfulness meditation can promote relaxation and improve overall well-being.

Skin Brushing: Dry skin brushing can stimulate the lymphatic system, promoting the removal of toxins from the body. Use a natural bristle brush to gently brush your skin in long, sweeping motions towards the heart. This practice can be done before showering and can help reduce symptoms of die-off reactions.

It's important to remember that while die-off reactions are uncomfortable, they are a temporary phase of the cleansing process. Being patient with yourself and allowing your body the time it needs to heal is essential. By implementing these strategies and supporting your body through the cleanse, you can reduce the severity of die-off reactions and make the process more manageable.

In summary, understanding die-off reactions and knowing how to manage them can make your parasite cleanse experience more effective and less daunting. By staying hydrated, supporting your liver, boosting your immune system, and incorporating supportive practices like detox baths, gentle exercise, and a nutrient-dense diet, you can navigate through this challenging phase with greater ease. Remember to listen to your body, monitor your symptoms, and seek professional guidance if needed. Your journey towards a parasite-free and healthier life is a significant step towards overall well-being.

IMMUNE SYSTEM SUPPORT

Supporting the immune system is vital during a parasite cleanse. As the body works hard to eliminate these unwelcome intruders, a robust immune response ensures that the process is efficient and that recovery is swift. There are several ways to bolster the immune system, from dietary supplements to stress reduction techniques. This section will delve into the most effective methods to keep your immune system functioning at its best.

Immune-Boosting Supplements

When it comes to boosting the immune system, certain supplements have been shown to be particularly effective. These supplements provide the body with essential nutrients that enhance immune function, making it easier to fight off infections and maintain overall health.

Vitamin C

Vitamin C is perhaps the most well-known immune-boosting supplement. It plays a crucial role in the production of white blood cells, which are essential for fighting infections. Additionally, vitamin C acts as an antioxidant, protecting the body from damage by free radicals. During a parasite cleanse, taking 500 to 1,000 mg of vitamin C daily can help strengthen your immune response.

Zinc

Zinc is another critical nutrient for immune function. It supports the development and function of immune cells and helps reduce inflammation. A deficiency in zinc can impair the immune system, making it harder to fend off infections. Supplementing with 15 to 30 mg of zinc daily can support your immune health during a cleanse.

Vitamin D

Vitamin D is essential for immune health, and many people have low levels, especially during the winter months. It enhances the pathogen-fighting effects of monocytes and macrophages, white blood cells that are important parts of the immune defense. Taking 1,000 to 2,000 IU of vitamin D daily can help maintain optimal immune function.

Probiotics

Probiotics are beneficial bacteria that support gut health. Since a significant portion of the immune system is located in the gut, maintaining a healthy gut flora is crucial for immune function. Probiotics can help balance the gut microbiome, making it easier for the body to fight off infections. Look for a probiotic supplement with multiple strains of bacteria and take it daily.

Echinacea

Echinacea is a popular herbal supplement known for its immune-boosting properties. It can enhance the activity of immune cells, helping the body to fight infections more effectively. Taking echinacea at the first sign of a die-off reaction or during the cleanse can support immune function. Typically, echinacea supplements are taken in doses of 300 to 500 mg, three times a day.

Elderberry

Elderberry is another powerful immune-boosting herb. It has been shown to reduce the duration and severity of colds and flu by enhancing immune function. Elderberry can be taken in syrup form, with a typical dose being 1 tablespoon of elderberry syrup, two to three times a day.

Garlic

Garlic has natural antimicrobial properties and can help support the immune system. It contains compounds that boost the disease-fighting response of some types of white blood cells. Fresh garlic can be added to meals, or garlic supplements can be taken to enhance immune function.

Turmeric

Turmeric contains curcumin, a compound with potent anti-inflammatory and antioxidant properties. It can help modulate the immune system, making it more efficient at fighting infections. Taking 500 to 1,000 mg of curcumin daily, with black pepper to enhance absorption, can support immune health.

Astragalus

Astragalus is an adaptogen herb known for its immune-boosting properties. It can enhance the body's resistance to stress and infections. Taking 500 to 1,000 mg of astragalus root extract daily can help support the immune system during a cleanse.

Medicinal Mushrooms

Medicinal mushrooms like reishi, shiitake, and maitake have immune-boosting properties. They contain beta-glucans, which enhance the activity of the immune system. Taking a mushroom supplement that contains a blend of these mushrooms can provide robust immune support.

Stress Reduction Techniques

The immune system can be significantly impacted by stress, which reduces its capacity to fend against illnesses. During a parasite cleanse, lowering stress is essential to preserving a robust immune system. Here are some effective stress reduction techniques:

Mindfulness Meditation

Mindfulness meditation entails focusing on and accepting the present moment without judgment. This technique can assist to reduce stress and boost immune function. Spend 10 to 20 minutes a day practicing mindfulness meditation. Find a peaceful spot to sit or lie down, close your eyes, and concentrate on your breathing. If your mind wanders, softly return your focus to your breathing.

Yoga

Yoga promotes relaxation and lowers stress levels by combining physical postures, breathing techniques, and meditation. Regular yoga practice helps strengthen the immune system and reduce stress hormones. Make it a point to do yoga several times a week for at least 20 to 30 minutes. All skill levels can find guided yoga sessions through a plethora of applications and web resources.

Deep Breathing Exercises

Exercises that involve deep breathing can help the body trigger its relaxation response, which lowers stress and boosts immunity. In a comfortable position, sit or lie down and practice deep breathing. Breathe in deeply with your nose, letting your belly expand, and then gently release the air through your mouth. For five to ten minutes, repeat this exercise while paying attention to your breathing.

Progressive Muscle Relaxation

Progressive muscle relaxation involves tensing and then relaxing different muscle groups in the body. This technique can help reduce stress and promote relaxation. Start by tensing the muscles in your toes for a few seconds, then relax them. Gradually work your way up the body, tensing and relaxing each muscle group.

Physical Activity

Regular physical activity can help reduce stress and boost immune function. Engage in moderate exercise like walking, jogging, swimming, or cycling for at least 30 minutes a day, most days of the week. Exercise helps reduce stress hormones and increases the production of endorphins, which improve mood and support immune health.

Adequate Sleep

Getting adequate sleep is critical for keeping a healthy immune system. Aim for 7-9 hours of sleep per night. Establish a consistent sleep schedule, develop a soothing nighttime routine, and make sure your sleeping environment is pleasant and distraction-free.

Creative Outlets

Engaging in creative activities like painting, drawing, writing, or playing a musical instrument can help reduce stress and promote relaxation. Find a creative outlet that you enjoy and make time for it regularly.

Social Connections

Maintaining strong social connections can help reduce stress and support immune function. Spend time with friends and family, whether in person or through virtual means. Talking with loved ones, sharing your experiences, and offering support can help alleviate stress.

Time in Nature

Spending time in nature can reduce stress and improve overall well-being. Take regular walks in a park, go hiking, or simply sit outside and enjoy the natural surroundings. Nature has a calming effect on the mind and body, which can support immune health.

Laughter and Joy

Laughter is a powerful stress reducer and can boost immune function. Watch a funny movie, read a humorous book, or spend time with people who make you laugh. Finding joy in everyday activities can have a positive impact on your health.

By incorporating these immune-boosting supplements and stress reduction techniques into your routine, you can support your immune system during a parasite cleanse. This holistic approach ensures that your body is well-equipped to handle the demands of the cleanse, promoting overall health and well-being. Remember, the goal is to create a balanced and sustainable lifestyle that supports your immune system and helps you achieve optimal health.

Conclusion

Navigating a parasite cleanse requires addressing both physical and emotional aspects. Managing die-off reactions is key to minimizing discomfort and staying committed to the process. Recognizing symptoms and applying strategies to ease them helps you stay on track.

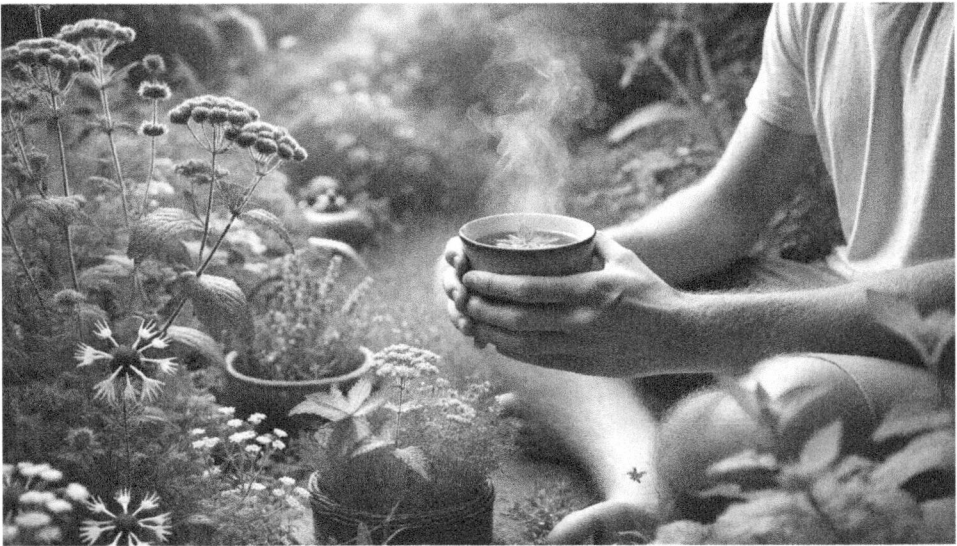

Supporting your immune system is equally important. Immune-boosting supplements and stress reduction techniques are essential both during the cleanse and for long-term health, helping to prevent future infections and maintain overall vitality.

This chapter provides you with practical advice and knowledge to manage the cleanse effectively. While some discomfort is natural, the right tools and mindset make it manageable. Be patient and kind to yourself throughout the process.

By combining effective management of die-off reactions with strong immune support, you enhance the cleanse's success and achieve lasting health benefits, turning the experience into a revitalizing and empowering journey.

8. Long-Term Parasite Cleanse and Prevention

Maintaining a parasite-free body is not just about undergoing a one-time cleanse; it's about adopting long-term habits and practices that support a healthy, resilient system. In this chapter, we delve into the essential strategies for ensuring that parasites do not take hold of your health again. We'll explore the critical role of diet and nutrition, the importance of regular cleansing routines, and the everyday hygiene practices that create a clean and safe environment. We also examine advanced natural prevention methods, from immune system support to the periodic use of herbs and supplements, which fortify the body against potential invasions.

The journey to long-term health involves more than just personal care; it extends to your lifestyle and environment. A clean home, mindful travel habits, and a proactive approach to reinfection prevention are all pivotal components of a comprehensive parasite defense strategy. By integrating these practices into your daily life, you can create a fortress of health that is resilient against parasites and other health threats.

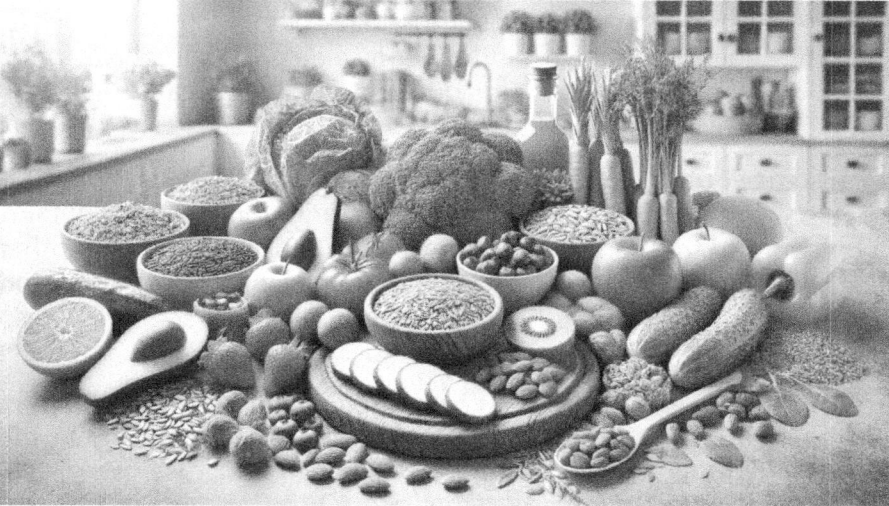

We also recognize that travel can introduce new challenges in maintaining a parasite-free body. Therefore, we provide practical advice for preparing your body before travel, essential items to carry, and maintaining safe hygiene practices while abroad. Our goal is to equip you with the knowledge and tools to stay healthy, no matter where life takes you.

MAINTAINING A PARASITE-FREE BODY

Achieving a parasite-free body is an accomplishment worth celebrating, but maintaining that state requires diligence and a proactive approach. The key to sustaining a parasite-free body lies in adopting healthy eating habits and establishing regular cleansing routines. These strategies not only help to prevent reinfestation but also support overall health and wellness.

Healthy Eating Habits

Diet plays a crucial role in maintaining a parasite-free body. A well-balanced diet rich in nutrients can strengthen the immune system, making it more resilient against parasitic infections. Emphasize foods that are known for their anti-parasitic properties and support gut health.

Fiber-Rich Foods: Consuming high-fiber foods helps in regular bowel movements, which is essential for flushing out toxins and any potential parasites. Include plenty of fruits, vegetables, whole grains, nuts, and seeds in your daily diet. Foods like apples, carrots, and chia seeds are excellent sources of fiber.

Probiotic-Rich Foods: Maintaining a healthy gut flora is vital for preventing parasite colonization. Incorporate probiotic-rich foods such as yogurt, kefir, sauerkraut, kimchi, and other fermented foods. These foods help promote a healthy balance of gut bacteria, which can inhibit the growth of harmful parasites.

Anti-Parasitic Foods: Certain foods have natural anti-parasitic properties and should be included regularly in your diet. Garlic, for instance, contains sulfur compounds that can help kill parasites. Pumpkin seeds are another excellent choice, as they contain cucurbitacin, which paralyzes worms and allows them to be eliminated from the body. Papaya seeds are also effective due to their high enzyme content.

Hydration: Staying well-hydrated is crucial for overall health and helps in flushing out toxins from the body. Drink plenty of water throughout the day. Herbal teas, especially those with anti-parasitic properties like wormwood and clove tea, can also be beneficial.

Avoiding Sugar and Processed Foods: Parasites thrive on sugar, so it is essential to limit or avoid foods high in sugar and processed ingredients. Opt for natural sweeteners like honey or maple syrup in moderation, and focus on whole, unprocessed foods.

Regular Cleansing Routines

Establishing regular cleansing routines helps ensure that your body remains free from parasites. Periodic detoxification can help in eliminating any parasites that might have been reintroduced into the body.

Daily Practices: Incorporate simple daily practices that support detoxification. Drinking warm lemon water first thing in the morning can help cleanse the liver and digestive system. Dry brushing your skin before a shower can stimulate lymphatic drainage and help in toxin removal.

Weekly Cleansing: Once a week, consider doing a gentle cleanse to support your body's natural detoxification processes. This could include a day of consuming only juices and smoothies made from anti-parasitic ingredients like ginger, turmeric, and cilantro. Alternatively, you can have a day where you eat only light, plant-based meals to give your digestive system a break.

Monthly Maintenance Cleanse: A more intensive cleanse can be done on a monthly basis. This might include fasting or consuming a specific anti-parasitic protocol for a few days. For instance, you can follow a regimen that includes taking herbal supplements such as black walnut hull, wormwood, and cloves, which are known for their efficacy in eliminating parasites.

Seasonal Detoxification: Every three to four months, perform a comprehensive detoxification program. This can align with the change of seasons and involve a more structured cleanse that includes dietary changes, herbal supplements, and other detox practices like sauna therapy or colon hydrotherapy.

Monitoring and Adjusting: Regularly monitor your health and be vigilant for any signs of parasitic infections. If you notice symptoms such as unexplained fatigue, digestive issues, or skin problems, consider revisiting your cleansing routine. Adjust your diet and detox practices as needed to maintain optimal health.

Maintaining a parasite-free body requires a combination of mindful eating and regular cleansing routines. By integrating these practices into your lifestyle, you not only protect yourself from parasitic infections but also enhance your overall health and well-being. Remember, consistency is key, and being proactive in your approach will help ensure long-term success in keeping parasites at bay.

HYGIENE AND LIFESTYLE

Maintaining a parasite-free life involves more than just dietary changes and regular cleanses; it requires a vigilant approach to hygiene and lifestyle. Creating a clean home environment and implementing strategies to prevent reinfections are essential steps to ensure long-term protection against parasites. This holistic approach not only guards against parasitic threats but also fosters a healthier, more harmonious living space.

Tips for a Clean Home Environment

A clean home environment is your first line of defense against parasites. Implementing thorough and regular cleaning routines can significantly reduce the risk of parasite infestation.

Regular Cleaning: Keep your living spaces clean and clutter-free. Regular vacuuming, dusting, and mopping can help eliminate parasites and their eggs. Pay special attention to high-traffic areas and places where pets frequent, as these are common hotspots for parasite activity.

Bedding and Upholstery: Wash bedding, curtains, and upholstered furniture covers in hot water regularly. Parasites, such as dust mites and fleas, can thrive in fabric. Using a high-temperature setting kills any parasites and their eggs. Consider using protective covers for mattresses and pillows to create an additional barrier.

Kitchen Hygiene: The kitchen can be a breeding ground for parasites if not maintained properly. Ensure all food is stored in airtight containers, and clean spills and crumbs immediately. Regularly disinfect countertops, cutting boards, and utensils. Be mindful of proper food handling practices to prevent cross-contamination.

Pet Care: If you have pets, they can be vectors for parasites. Regularly bathe and groom your pets, and ensure they receive routine veterinary care, including parasite prevention treatments. Clean pet bedding frequently and keep their living areas sanitary.

Natural Cleaning Agents: Opt for natural cleaning agents like vinegar, baking soda, and essential oils (such as tea tree or eucalyptus oil) that have antimicrobial properties. These not only help in cleaning but also deter parasites from settling in your home.

Ventilation and Sunlight: Ensure your home is well-ventilated and receives plenty of sunlight. Fresh air and sunlight create an inhospitable environment for many parasites. Open windows regularly and use fans to circulate air, reducing humidity levels that can attract parasites.

Preventing Reinfections

Preventing reinfections requires a proactive approach that extends beyond the home. It involves personal hygiene, regular health checks, and maintaining a conscious effort to avoid environments where parasites thrive.

Personal Hygiene: Regular handwashing with soap and water is one of the simplest and most effective ways to prevent parasite transmission. Wash your hands thoroughly after using the bathroom, before preparing or eating food, and after handling pets. Encourage good hygiene practices among family members, especially children.

Safe Food Practices: Always wash fruits and vegetables thoroughly before consumption. Cook meat to the appropriate temperatures to kill any parasites that might be present. Avoid consuming raw or undercooked seafood and meat, as these are common sources of parasites.

Water Safety: Ensure your drinking water is clean and safe. Use a water filter if necessary, and avoid drinking untreated water from natural sources such as rivers or lakes. When traveling, be cautious about the local water quality and prefer bottled or boiled water.

Travel Precautions: When traveling, especially to regions with higher risks of parasitic infections, take extra precautions. Use insect repellent, wear protective clothing, and avoid walking barefoot in areas where parasites are known to be prevalent. Be mindful of food and water safety, and consider pre-travel consultations for appropriate preventive measures.

Regular Health Checks: Schedule regular health check-ups to monitor for any signs of parasitic infections. Early detection and treatment can prevent more severe health issues. Discuss any unusual symptoms with your healthcare provider and consider periodic stool tests to ensure no parasites are present.

Clothing and Footwear: Wear protective clothing and footwear when walking in areas where parasites are common, such as forests or grasslands. Parasites like ticks and fleas can latch onto your clothing and find their way into your home. After spending time outdoors, check your body and clothing for any unwanted hitchhikers.

Household Practices: Implement household rules to prevent parasites from gaining a foothold. For instance, establish a no-shoes policy inside the house to avoid bringing in contaminants from outside. Encourage the use of separate indoor and outdoor footwear to minimize the risk of parasite transmission.

By incorporating these hygiene and lifestyle practices, you can create a robust defense against parasites and ensure a healthier living environment. These measures not only protect you and your family but also promote a sense of well-being and peace of mind. Adopting these habits as part of your daily routine can significantly reduce the risk of parasite-related issues, allowing you to enjoy a parasite-free life with confidence.

ADVANCED NATURAL PREVENTION

Maintaining a parasite-free lifestyle extends beyond immediate cleanses and routine hygiene; it involves a comprehensive approach to strengthen the body's natural defenses and implement long-term preventive strategies. Advanced natural prevention focuses on bolstering the immune system, adhering to an anti-parasitic diet, utilizing herbs and supplements proactively, and incorporating periodic detoxification techniques.

Strengthening the Immune System Naturally

A robust immune system is your first line of defense against parasitic infections. Strengthening it through natural means ensures that your body is better equipped to fend off parasitic threats.

Nutrient-Rich Diet: Consuming a diet rich in essential nutrients supports immune function. Incorporate plenty of fruits and vegetables, particularly those high in vitamins C and E, zinc, and beta-carotene. Foods such as citrus fruits, berries, spinach, and nuts are excellent choices.

Probiotics: Maintaining a healthy gut flora is crucial for immune health. Probiotic-rich foods like yogurt, kefir, sauerkraut, and kimchi help balance the gut microbiome, which plays a vital role in immune function.

Regular Exercise: Engaging in regular physical activity enhances circulation, reduces inflammation, and supports overall immune health. Aim for at least 30 minutes of moderate exercise most days of the week.

Adequate Sleep: Quality sleep is essential for immune function. Ensure you get 7-9 hours of uninterrupted sleep each night to allow your body to repair and strengthen its defenses.

Hydration: Staying well-hydrated is key to maintaining a healthy immune system. Drink plenty of water throughout the day to help your body flush out toxins and support overall bodily functions.

Stress Management: Chronic stress weakens the immune system. Incorporate stress-reducing practices such as meditation, deep breathing exercises, and yoga to maintain emotional and physical health.

Long-Term Anti-Parasitic Diet

Adopting a long-term anti-parasitic diet helps prevent infections and supports overall health. This diet focuses on foods that create an inhospitable environment for parasites.

Garlic and Onions: Both garlic and onions contain sulfur compounds with natural anti-parasitic properties. Including them in your daily meals can help deter parasites.

Pumpkin Seeds: Rich in cucurbitacin, pumpkin seeds are effective against intestinal parasites. Snack on a handful daily or add them to salads and smoothies.

Papaya Seeds: Known for their anti-parasitic properties, papaya seeds can be consumed in smoothies or dried and ground into a powder.

Pineapple: Bromelain, an enzyme found in pineapple, has anti-parasitic effects. Enjoy fresh pineapple or drink pineapple juice regularly.

Carrots: High in beta-carotene, carrots support immune function and help combat parasites. Eat them raw, juiced, or cooked.

Fermented Foods: Foods like kimchi, sauerkraut, and kombucha support gut health and provide an environment that discourages parasites.

Herbs and Spices: Incorporate anti-parasitic herbs and spices such as turmeric, ginger, cayenne pepper, and oregano into your diet. These not only add flavor but also boost your body's defenses.

Preventive Use of Herbs and Supplements

Certain herbs and supplements can be used preventively to maintain a parasite-free body. These natural remedies support overall health and create a hostile environment for parasites.

Wormwood and Black Walnut: Both are potent anti-parasitic herbs. Taking them in tincture or capsule form can help prevent infections.

Cloves: Known for their ability to kill parasite eggs, cloves can be taken as a supplement or added to teas and foods.

Neem: With its broad-spectrum anti-parasitic properties, neem can be used as a supplement or in herbal teas.

Oregano Oil: A powerful natural antibiotic and anti-parasitic, oregano oil can be taken in capsule form or added to food.

Probiotics: Regular use of probiotic supplements supports gut health and immunity, creating an environment unfavorable to parasites.

Vitamin C and Zinc: Both are essential for immune function. Consider taking them as supplements if your diet is lacking.

Periodic Detoxification Techniques

Regular detoxification helps to eliminate any parasites that may have entered your system and supports overall health.

Herbal Cleanses: Periodic herbal cleanses using combinations of anti-parasitic herbs like wormwood, black walnut, and clove can help keep your body parasite-free.

Juice Fasting: Short-term juice fasting with anti-parasitic juices, such as those containing papaya and pineapple, can help cleanse your system.

Colon Cleansing: Using natural methods like water enemas or herbal colon cleanses periodically can help eliminate parasites and their eggs from the intestines.

Liver Cleanses: Supporting liver health through specific cleanses using herbs like milk thistle and dandelion root helps the body detoxify effectively.

By integrating these advanced natural prevention strategies into your lifestyle, you can create a strong, resilient body capable of defending against parasites. These measures not only protect against immediate threats but also promote long-term health and well-being, ensuring that you remain parasite-free and vibrant.

ADVICE FOR TRAVELERS

Traveling can expose you to a variety of environments and conditions that increase the risk of parasitic infections. By preparing adequately and adopting certain practices, you can protect yourself and enjoy your travels without compromising your health. Here are some essential tips and strategies for maintaining a parasite-free state while on the go.

Natural Preparation Before Travel

Before starting your cleanse, it's essential to boost your body's natural defenses and prepare for potential parasite exposure. This preparation will help your body handle the cleansing process more effectively and protect against future infections.

Boost Your Immune System: Begin a regimen of immune-boosting supplements at least two weeks before departure. Consider taking vitamin C, zinc, and probiotics to enhance your body's natural defenses.

Start a Gentle Cleanse: A week before traveling, initiate a gentle parasite cleanse using natural remedies like garlic, pumpkin seeds, and papaya seeds. This can help to rid your body of any existing parasites and create an inhospitable environment for new ones.

Hydrate and Nourish: Ensure you are well-hydrated and consuming a nutrient-rich diet. Focus on foods high in antioxidants, vitamins, and minerals to fortify your immune system.

Pack a Health Kit: Prepare a travel health kit that includes essential items such as hand sanitizer, disinfectant wipes, a water purifier or tablets, and a first-aid kit. Include any necessary medications and natural supplements you may need.

Herbs and Supplements to Carry While Traveling

Certain herbs and supplements can provide an additional layer of protection against parasites during your travels. Carry these natural remedies in your travel kit for preventive use and immediate response if needed.

Black Walnut and Wormwood: These powerful anti-parasitic herbs can be taken in capsule or tincture form. Use them preventively or at the first sign of an infection.

Oregano Oil: Known for its broad-spectrum antimicrobial properties, oregano oil can be taken in capsules or added to water to combat parasites.

Grapefruit Seed Extract: This extract has potent anti-parasitic and antibacterial properties. It can be used as a preventive measure or to treat symptoms that arise.

Activated Charcoal: Useful for binding toxins and helping the body eliminate them, activated charcoal can be taken if you suspect you have ingested contaminated food or water.

Probiotics: Maintain your gut health by taking probiotics daily. They support a balanced gut flora, which is essential for immune function and overall health.

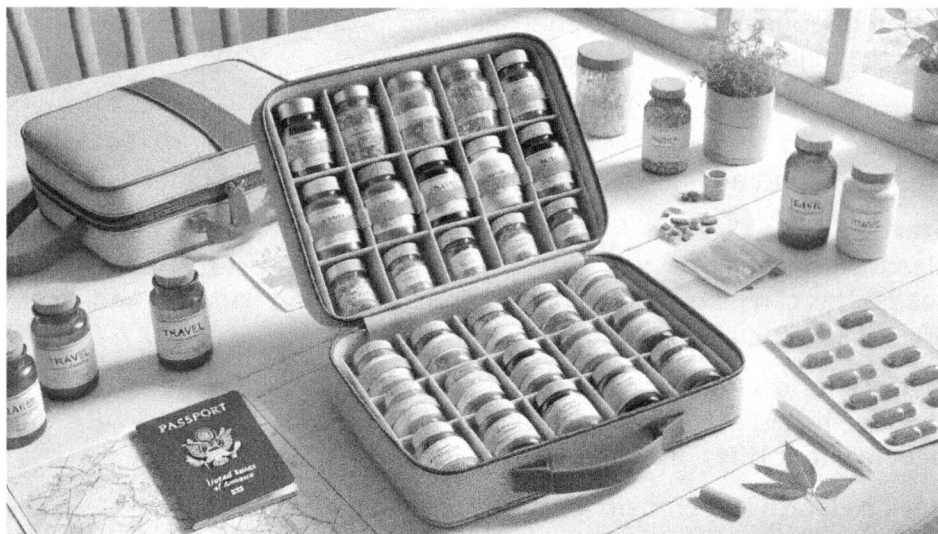

Hygiene Practices During Travel

Maintaining strict hygiene practices is critical in preventing parasitic infections while traveling, especially in regions where sanitation may be compromised.

Hand Hygiene: Always wash your hands with soap and water before eating and after using the restroom. When soap and water are not available, use a hand sanitizer with at least 60% alcohol content.

Food Safety: Be cautious about what and where you eat. Opt for hot, freshly cooked foods and avoid raw or undercooked meats, seafood, and unwashed fruits and vegetables. Peel fruits yourself and avoid salads or foods that may have been washed in contaminated water.

Water Safety: Drink bottled or purified water. Avoid ice cubes and beverages made with tap water. Consider using a portable water purifier or water purification tablets.

Personal Items: Avoid sharing personal items such as towels, razors, and toothbrushes. Use your own toiletries to minimize the risk of cross-contamination.

Footwear: Wear shoes, especially in areas where parasites like hookworms are prevalent. Avoid walking barefoot on soil or sand.

Managing Diet in High-Risk Countries

Adhering to a safe diet while traveling in high-risk areas can significantly reduce your risk of parasitic infections.

Stick to Cooked Foods: Prefer hot, thoroughly cooked meals over raw or cold dishes. Boiling and steaming are effective methods to kill parasites and their eggs.

Avoid Street Food: While street food can be tempting, it often carries a higher risk of contamination. Choose restaurants with good hygiene practices instead.

Bottled Beverages: Drink bottled or canned beverages. Avoid drinks that may be made with tap water or unpasteurized dairy products.

Clean Produce: If you buy fresh produce, clean it thoroughly with purified water. Alternatively, choose fruits and vegetables that can be peeled or cooked.

Post-Travel Natural Cleansing

After returning from your travels, it's wise to undergo a natural cleansing regimen to eliminate any potential parasites you may have been exposed to.

Resume Your Cleanse: Reinitiate a parasite cleanse using herbs like wormwood, black walnut, and cloves. Follow a structured regimen to ensure any parasites are effectively eradicated.

Hydration and Detox: Drink plenty of purified water and incorporate detoxifying foods like garlic, ginger, and turmeric into your diet. These help to cleanse your system and support your liver in detoxification.

Probiotics: Continue taking probiotics to maintain gut health and support your immune system.

Monitor Symptoms: Pay attention to any unusual symptoms such as digestive issues, fatigue, or skin rashes. If symptoms persist, consult a healthcare professional for further evaluation.

By implementing these strategies, you can safeguard your health while traveling and enjoy your adventures with peace of mind.

Conclusion

Living parasite-free requires ongoing commitment to healthy habits. Advanced strategies like immune-boosting and using herbs further strengthen your defenses. Periodic detoxification maintains resilience. These practices not only prevent parasites but enhance overall health.

9. Parasite Cleanse for Children and Pets

Parasites can affect every member of the family, including children and pets. Recognizing and addressing these issues promptly is essential for maintaining overall health and well-being. Children, with their developing immune systems and frequent close contact with the ground and animals, are particularly vulnerable to parasitic infections. Similarly, pets, whether they spend most of their time indoors or outdoors, are prone to a variety of parasites that can easily transfer to humans. Understanding how to identify symptoms, safely cleanse, and maintain a parasite-free environment is crucial for both children and pets. This chapter delves into the specific symptoms to watch for in children and pets, natural cleansing methods that are safe and effective, and dietary strategies that support long-term health and prevention. By taking a proactive approach to managing parasites, you can protect the most vulnerable members of your household from the discomfort and health risks associated with parasitic infections. The following sections will provide detailed guidance on how to achieve and maintain a parasite-free state for children and pets, using natural and holistic methods that support their overall health and well-being.

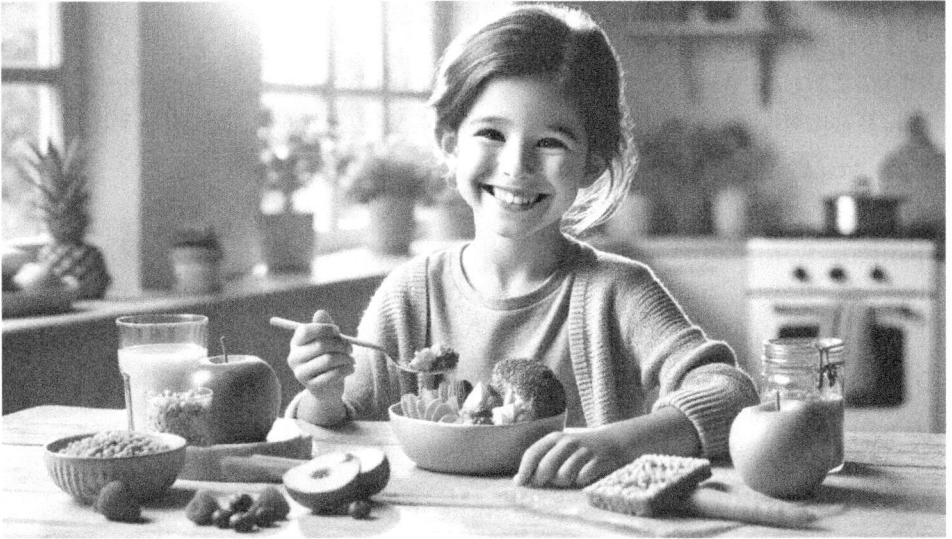

PARASITE CLEANSE FOR CHILDREN

Children are particularly vulnerable to parasitic infections due to their developing immune systems and their tendency to explore their environments with less caution. Understanding the specific symptoms of parasitic infections in children and employing safe, natural methods for cleansing can significantly improve their health and well-being. Ensuring that their diet supports a parasite-free body is also crucial.

Specific Symptoms in Children

Parasitic infections in children often present differently than in adults. Some common symptoms to look out for include:

Gastrointestinal Issues: Persistent diarrhea, stomach cramps, bloating, and gas can indicate a parasitic infection. Children may also experience frequent nausea and vomiting.

Weight Loss and Poor Appetite: An unexplained drop in weight or a significant loss of appetite may signal the presence of parasites.

Fatigue and Weakness: Parasites can drain essential nutrients from the body, leading to chronic fatigue and general weakness.

Skin Irritations: Rashes, itching, and hives can be signs of a parasitic infection. In some cases, children might develop eczema-like symptoms.

Behavioral Changes: Irritability, restlessness, and difficulty concentrating can occur as a result of parasitic infections. Nighttime teeth grinding (bruxism) is also a common symptom.

Anal Itching: Pinworms, one of the most common parasites in children, often cause intense itching around the anus, particularly at night.

Safe and Natural Methods for Kids

When dealing with parasitic infections in children, it is crucial to use gentle and safe methods. Here are some effective natural remedies:

Garlic: Known for its antiparasitic properties, garlic can be a powerful ally. Crush a clove of garlic and mix it with honey to make it more palatable for children. Ensure they consume it on an empty stomach for maximum effectiveness.

Papaya Seeds: These seeds are potent in eliminating parasites. Blend a teaspoon of dried papaya seeds into a smoothie or mix them with honey for a more child-friendly option.

Pumpkin Seeds: Rich in cucurbitacin, which paralyzes parasites, pumpkin seeds can be given as a snack or blended into smoothies.

Coconut Oil: Coconut oil has antiparasitic effects and can be added to the child's diet. Start with a small amount, such as a teaspoon, and gradually increase.

Probiotics: A healthy gut flora is essential for combating parasites. Include probiotic-rich foods like yogurt, kefir, and fermented vegetables in the child's diet.

Herbal Teas: Mild herbal teas such as chamomile or ginger can soothe the digestive system and help eliminate parasites. Ensure the teas are not too strong for young children.

Diet and Nutrition for Children

A well-balanced diet plays a crucial role in preventing and managing parasitic infections in children by strengthening their immune system and creating an environment that is less hospitable to parasites. Here are some essential dietary guidelines to follow:

High-Fiber Foods: Fiber is key to cleansing the digestive tract and naturally eliminating parasites from the body. Include a variety of fiber-rich fruits, vegetables, and whole grains in your child's diet to promote a healthy digestive system.

Low-Sugar Diet: Parasites thrive on sugar. Reducing sugar intake can help starve the parasites and support the child's immune system.

Hydration: Ensure the child drinks plenty of water throughout the day to help flush out toxins and parasites.

Antiparasitic Foods: Incorporate foods known for their antiparasitic properties, such as garlic, onions, ginger, turmeric, and cloves, into meals.

Healthy Fats: Healthy fats from sources like avocados, nuts, seeds, and coconut oil can support the immune system and aid in the absorption of fat-soluble vitamins.

Fermented Foods: Fermented foods like sauerkraut, kimchi, and kefir are excellent for maintaining a healthy gut flora, which is essential in fighting off parasites.

Protein-Rich Foods: Ensure your child receives adequate protein from lean meats, fish, eggs, legumes, and nuts. Protein is crucial for growth, development, and maintaining a strong immune system, which is vital for resisting infections of all kinds, including parasitic ones.

Example Meal Plan for Children

Here is a sample meal plan that incorporates these dietary guidelines:

BREAKFAST

o   Smoothie made with banana, spinach, papaya seeds, and almond milk.
o   Whole-grain toast with avocado and a sprinkle of pumpkin seeds.

MID-MORNING SNACK

o   Apple slices with a teaspoon of coconut oil drizzled on top.
o   A small serving of yogurt with a handful of berries.

LUNCH

o   Quinoa salad with chopped vegetables, chickpeas, and a lemon-garlic dressing.
o   A side of fermented vegetables, such as sauerkraut.

AFTERNOON SNACK

o   Carrot sticks with hummus.
o   A small bowl of mixed nuts and seeds.

DINNER

o   Baked chicken seasoned with turmeric and ginger, served with steamed broccoli and sweet potatoes.
o   A cup of mild chamomile tea.

BEDTIME

o   A glass of warm milk with a pinch of turmeric and honey.

Conclusion

Managing parasitic infections in children requires a balanced approach focusing on safety and effectiveness. Recognizing specific symptoms allows for early intervention. Safe, natural methods can provide gentle yet effective treatment. A supportive diet is crucial for long-term prevention.

This section outlines natural strategies to combat parasites in children, addressing current infections and building future immunity. Incorporating these practices into your child's routine can promote optimal health and resilience against parasites.

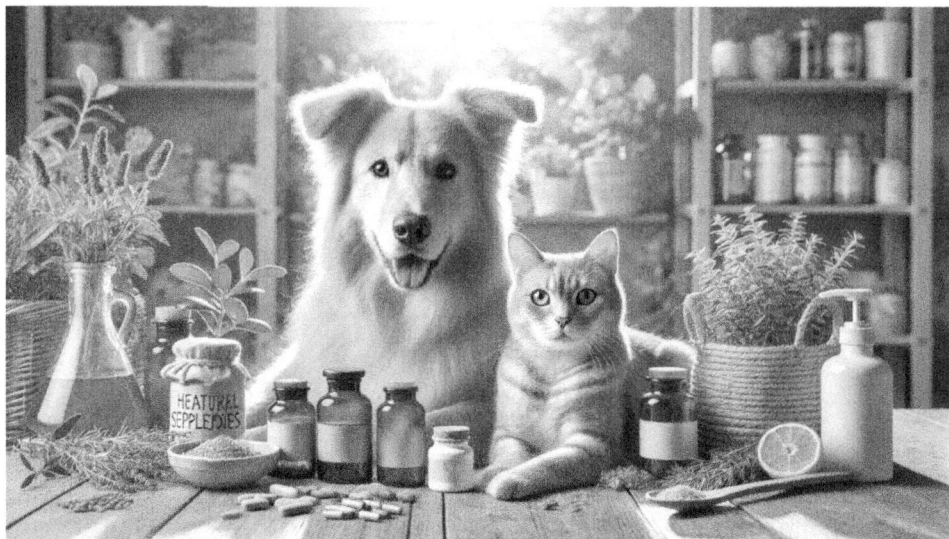

PARASITE CLEANSE FOR PETS

Pets are beloved members of many families, and their health is just as important as our own. Parasitic infections in pets, particularly dogs and cats, are common and can significantly impact their well-being. Understanding the symptoms and diagnosis of parasitic infections in pets, implementing natural cleansing methods, and taking preventive measures are crucial steps in maintaining their health.

Symptoms and Diagnosis in Dogs and Cats

Parasitic infections in pets can manifest in various ways. Recognizing the signs and seeking prompt diagnosis can help ensure effective treatment.

COMMON SYMPTOMS

Gastrointestinal Distress: Similar to humans, pets with parasitic infections often exhibit symptoms like diarrhea, vomiting, and loss of appetite. Persistent or recurring gastrointestinal issues should be a red flag.

Weight Loss: Unexplained weight loss, despite a normal or increased appetite, can indicate a parasitic infection. Parasites compete for nutrients, leaving pets malnourished.

Lethargy: A sudden decrease in energy levels or overall lethargy is a common symptom. Pets may seem less interested in activities they usually enjoy.

Skin Irritations: Parasites like fleas and mites cause severe itching, leading to excessive scratching, hair loss, and skin infections. Pets may also develop rashes or hives.

Scooting and Licking: Dogs, in particular, may drag their rear ends on the ground or lick their anal areas excessively, indicating irritation from parasites like tapeworms or roundworms.

Coughing and Respiratory Issues: Heartworms, a severe parasitic infection, can cause coughing, difficulty breathing, and exercise intolerance in dogs.

DIAGNOSIS

Fecal Examination: A vet can analyze a stool sample to identify the presence of eggs, larvae, or adult parasites. This is one of the most common diagnostic methods.

Blood Tests: Blood tests can detect specific parasites, such as heartworms, and evaluate the overall health impact on the pet.

Physical Examination: A thorough physical examination by a veterinarian can reveal signs of parasitic infections, such as skin lesions, abdominal distention, and respiratory abnormalities.

Imaging Techniques: In some cases, imaging techniques like X-rays or ultrasounds may be used to identify internal parasites.

Natural Cleansing Methods for Pets

Using natural methods to cleanse pets of parasites can be effective and gentle, avoiding the potential side effects of chemical treatments. Here are some proven natural remedies:

Diatomaceous Earth: Food-grade diatomaceous earth can be added to pet food to help eliminate internal parasites. It works by dehydrating and killing the parasites without harming the pet. The recommended dosage is 1 teaspoon per day for small dogs and cats and up to 1 tablespoon for larger dogs.

Pumpkin Seeds: Pumpkin seeds contain cucurbitacin, which paralyzes parasites and helps expel them from the digestive tract. Ground pumpkin seeds can be mixed into the pet's food—approximately 1 teaspoon for small pets and up to 1 tablespoon for larger pets.

Garlic: While garlic is controversial and should be used with caution, it can help repel parasites in small, controlled doses. Consult a veterinarian before using garlic, as it can be toxic in large amounts. Typically, a small amount of fresh garlic (half a clove) can be mixed into the pet's food once a week.

Apple Cider Vinegar: Adding a small amount of apple cider vinegar to your pet's water can create an environment that is hostile to parasites. Use about 1 teaspoon per quart of water.

Herbal Teas: Mild herbal teas, such as chamomile or ginger, can be given to pets to soothe the digestive system and help expel parasites. Ensure the tea is not too strong and is cooled before offering it to your pet.

Coconut Oil: Coconut oil has antiparasitic properties and can be added to your pet's diet. Start with a small amount (1/4 teaspoon for small pets and 1 teaspoon for larger pets) and gradually increase.

Prevention and Maintenance of Pet Health

Preventing parasitic infections and maintaining overall health involves a combination of good hygiene practices, regular check-ups, and a balanced diet.

HYGIENE PRACTICES

Regular Grooming: Regular brushing and bathing help keep the pet's coat clean and free of parasites. Use natural, pet-safe shampoos that contain antiparasitic ingredients like neem or eucalyptus.

Clean Living Environment: Keep the pet's living area clean by regularly washing bedding, toys, and bowls. Vacuum carpets and upholstery frequently to remove any parasite eggs or larvae.

Flea and Tick Control: Use natural flea and tick repellents, such as essential oils like lavender, eucalyptus, and citronella. Always dilute essential oils and consult a vet before applying them to pets.

Proper Waste Disposal: Dispose of pet waste promptly and properly. Parasite eggs can contaminate the soil and spread to other animals and humans.

REGULAR CHECK-UPS

Veterinary Visits: Regular check-ups with a veterinarian are essential. Annual fecal exams and blood tests can detect early signs of parasitic infections.

Deworming: Follow a regular deworming schedule as recommended by your veterinarian, especially for young animals.

BALANCED DIET

Nutrient-Rich Foods: Provide a balanced diet rich in nutrients to support your pet's immune system. High-quality commercial pet foods or homemade diets should include proteins, fats, vitamins, and minerals.

Probiotics: Adding probiotics to your pet's diet can support gut health and improve resistance to parasites. Probiotic supplements or foods like yogurt (in small amounts) can be beneficial.

Hydration: Ensure your pet has access to fresh, clean water at all times. Proper hydration supports overall health and helps flush out toxins.

By incorporating these natural methods and preventive measures, you can help your pets maintain a parasite-free and healthy life. Regular monitoring, good hygiene, and a balanced diet are the cornerstones of effective parasite management for your furry friends.

Conclusion

Protecting children and pets from parasites requires vigilance and knowledge. By recognizing specific symptoms and using safe, natural cleansing methods, you can effectively safeguard your family's most vulnerable members.

For children, focus on immune-boosting foods and gentle natural remedies. For pets, regular check-ups, proper grooming, and natural antiparasitic supplements are key.

Maintain a clean environment and practice good hygiene to reduce reinfection risks. Regular monitoring and a balanced diet form the foundation of a parasite-free household.

With these strategies, you're well-equipped to tackle parasites and ensure the health and happiness of your entire family, including your furry friends.

10. Understanding and Managing External Parasites

External parasites like fleas, ticks, lice, and mites pose significant threats to both human and pet health, causing discomfort and spreading diseases such as Lyme disease and scabies. Effective management of these pests requires early detection, accurate identification, and proper treatment.

This chapter covers the identification, symptoms, and natural treatment methods for common external parasites, as well as long-term prevention strategies to maintain a parasite-free environment. By understanding their habits and life cycles, you can protect your home and loved ones more effectively, ensuring a healthier living space.

TYPES OF EXTERNAL PARASITES

External parasites are organisms that live on the surface of their host, deriving their nutrition directly from the host's blood or skin. These parasites can cause significant discomfort and health issues for both humans and animals. Understanding the types of external parasites is crucial for effective management and prevention. Here, we will explore four common types: fleas, ticks, lice, and mites (scabies).

Fleas

Fleas are small, wingless insects that are highly adept at jumping. They feed on the blood of mammals and birds, making them a common nuisance for pets and humans alike. Fleas are reddish-brown and typically measure 1 to 3 millimeters in length. Despite their small size, they can cause severe itching and discomfort due to their bites. Flea bites can lead to allergic reactions and secondary infections from scratching.

Fleas have a complex life cycle that includes eggs, larvae, pupae, and adults. They reproduce rapidly, and a single female flea can lay up to 50 eggs per day. These eggs can fall off the host and develop in the surrounding environment, making it challenging to control an infestation. Fleas are also known vectors for diseases such as the bubonic plague and typhus.

Ticks

Ticks are arachnids, closely related to spiders and mites. They are external parasites that attach themselves to the skin of their hosts to feed on blood. Ticks vary in size from 3 to 5 millimeters and can swell significantly when engorged with blood. They are typically found in grassy, wooded areas and are most active during warm months.

Ticks pose a significant health risk because they can transmit serious diseases, such as Lyme disease, Rocky Mountain spotted fever, and tularemia. Ticks go through four life stages: egg, larva, nymph, and adult. Each stage requires a blood meal to progress to the next. Ticks can attach to any part of the body but are commonly found in hidden areas such as the scalp, armpits, and groin.

Lice

Lice are small, wingless insects that live on the skin and hair of their hosts. There are three main types of lice that affect humans: head lice, body lice, and pubic lice (crabs). Head lice are the most common and are primarily found on the scalp. Lice are about the size of a sesame seed and can be gray or brown. They feed on human blood several times a day, which can cause intense itching and irritation.

Lice spread through direct contact with an infested person or through sharing personal items such as hats, combs, and bedding. Lice eggs, known as nits, are attached to the hair shaft and can be difficult to remove. Lice infestations, while not dangerous, can lead to secondary infections from scratching and are often considered a significant social stigma.

Mites (Scabies)

Scabies is caused by a specific type of mite known as Sarcoptes scabiei. These microscopic mites burrow into the skin to lay their eggs, causing intense itching and a rash that can resemble pimples or blisters. The itching is often worse at night and can lead to severe discomfort and sleep disturbances.

Scabies is highly contagious and spreads through close personal contact or sharing of bedding, clothing, and other personal items. The mites can live on the skin for 1 to 2 months, during which they continue to reproduce and exacerbate the infestation. While scabies itself does not transmit diseases, the intense scratching can lead to skin infections.

SYMPTOMS AND IDENTIFICATION

Identifying external parasitic infections promptly is essential for effective treatment and prevention of further spread. Recognizing the signs and knowing the appropriate diagnostic techniques can make a significant difference in managing these pests. Here, we delve into the symptoms and identification methods for the four main types of external parasites: fleas, ticks, lice, and mites (scabies).

Signs of External Parasitic Infections

Fleas: Flea infestations are characterized by several telltale signs. The most obvious symptom is intense itching and scratching, particularly around the neck, behind the ears, and at the base of the tail in pets. In humans, flea bites often appear as small, red bumps that may be surrounded by a halo. These bites are commonly found on the ankles and legs. Flea dirt, which looks like tiny black pepper grains, is another clear indication. This "dirt" is actually flea feces and can be found in the fur of pets or on bedding.

Ticks: Tick bites are often painless, which makes these parasites particularly insidious. The primary sign of a tick bite is the presence of the tick itself, attached to the skin. Inflammation and redness around the bite site are common, and in some cases, a rash may develop. One distinctive symptom to watch for is a bullseye-shaped rash, which can be indicative of Lyme disease, a serious condition transmitted by ticks. Additional symptoms may include fever, fatigue, and muscle aches, which warrant immediate medical attention.

Lice: Lice infestations are accompanied by persistent itching, particularly on the scalp, neck, and behind the ears. For body lice, itching and irritation may be widespread across the body, especially where clothing seams contact the skin. Nits, or lice eggs, can be seen attached to hair shafts close to the scalp. These tiny, oval-shaped eggs are usually white or yellowish and can be difficult to remove. Lice themselves are tiny, about the size of a sesame seed, and can be seen moving in the hair.

Mites (Scabies): Scabies mites burrow into the skin, causing intense itching, especially at night. This itching is often accompanied by a rash that can appear as small red bumps, blisters, or pimple-like eruptions. The burrows themselves may be visible as thin, wavy, grayish lines on the skin, typically found in the webbing between the fingers, on the wrists, elbows, and around the waist. The itching and rash are a result of the body's allergic reaction to the mites and their waste.

Diagnostic Techniques

Fleas: Diagnosing a flea infestation can often be done visually. Checking pets thoroughly by parting their fur and looking for fleas or flea dirt is the first step. Using a flea comb can help to catch fleas and remove flea dirt from the fur. In severe cases, veterinarians may perform a skin test to rule out other causes of itching and irritation.

Ticks: Ticks are usually found through careful inspection of the body, focusing on areas such as the scalp, armpits, groin, and behind the knees.

Once a tick is found, it should be carefully removed with tweezers, ensuring the entire tick is extracted. Blood tests may be necessary if a tick bite is suspected to have transmitted a disease, such as Lyme disease.

Lice: Lice and nits are visible to the naked eye but can be more easily identified using a fine-toothed comb. Combing through wet or damp hair can help dislodge nits and lice. If lice are suspected, it is advisable to check the hair in sections under bright light. For body lice, checking seams of clothing and bedding for lice or their eggs is necessary. In some cases, magnification or a microscope may be used for confirmation.

Mites (Scabies): Diagnosing scabies involves a thorough examination of the skin. A healthcare provider may look for characteristic burrows and take a skin scraping to examine under a microscope. The presence of mites, eggs, or mite feces in the scraping confirms scabies. Given the intense itching and potential for widespread infestation, prompt and accurate diagnosis is essential.

Understanding the symptoms and utilizing the appropriate diagnostic techniques are critical steps in managing external parasitic infections effectively. By identifying these parasites early, you can take the necessary measures to treat and prevent further infestations, ensuring a healthier environment for both humans and pets.

NATURAL TREATMENTS FOR EXTERNAL PARASITES

When it comes to managing external parasites, natural treatments can offer effective and gentle alternatives to chemical-based solutions. Utilizing herbal sprays, essential oils, and other natural preventative measures can help to mitigate infestations without the harsh side effects that often accompany conventional treatments. Here's a detailed look at some of the best natural treatments for fleas, ticks, lice, and mites.

Herbal Sprays and Washes

Herbal Sprays Herbal sprays are a fantastic way to keep external parasites at bay. These sprays can be made at home using ingredients like lavender, eucalyptus, and rosemary, which are known for their repellent properties. To create an effective herbal spray, steep a mixture of these herbs in boiling water, let it cool, and then strain the liquid into a spray bottle. Spritz the solution on pet fur, bedding, and other areas where parasites may reside. Regular application can deter fleas, ticks, and lice from taking hold.

Herbal Washes Herbal washes can be used during baths to help repel and eliminate parasites. A common recipe includes a combination of neem leaves and peppermint. Boil neem leaves in water, add a few drops of peppermint essential oil, and let the mixture cool. Use this herbal wash as a final rinse after your pet's regular bath. Neem is especially effective due to its natural insecticidal properties, which can kill and repel parasites.

Essential Oils for Topical Use

Essential oils are potent natural remedies for external parasites. However, they must be used with caution, especially on pets, to avoid irritation or toxicity. Here are some of the most effective essential oils and how to use them:

Lavender Oil Lavender oil is well-known for its calming properties, but it also works as a powerful insect repellent. Mix a few drops of lavender oil with a carrier oil like coconut or olive oil and apply it to the back of your pet's neck or around the ears. This mixture can also be added to your pet's shampoo for an anti-parasitic wash.

Tea Tree Oil Tea tree oil has strong antifungal and antibacterial properties, making it an excellent treatment for lice and mites. However, tea tree oil should be heavily diluted before use. A safe ratio is one drop of tea tree oil per tablespoon of carrier oil. Apply the mixture to the affected areas, being careful to avoid sensitive regions like the eyes and mucous membranes.

Eucalyptus Oil Eucalyptus oil is another effective repellent for fleas and ticks. A diluted mixture can be sprayed on bedding and around the home to deter these pests. Additionally, adding a few drops to a pet's collar can provide ongoing protection.

Natural Preventative Measures

Prevention is always better than cure, and there are several natural strategies you can employ to keep external parasites from becoming a problem in the first place.

Regular Grooming Regular grooming is crucial for detecting and removing parasites before they become a significant issue. Use a fine-toothed comb to check for fleas, lice, and ticks. Bathing your pets with natural shampoos that contain anti-parasitic herbs like neem and eucalyptus can help keep their skin and coat parasite-free.

Environmental Control Maintaining a clean environment is essential for preventing parasite infestations. Regularly wash your pet's bedding, vacuum your home frequently, and consider using natural flea powders made from diatomaceous earth around your home. Diatomaceous earth is a non-toxic powder that dehydrates and kills insects but is safe for pets and humans when used correctly.

Diet and Nutrition A healthy diet can strengthen your pet's immune system, making them less attractive to parasites. Incorporate foods rich in essential fatty acids, such as fish oil or flaxseed oil, into their diet. These can improve skin health and create an environment that is less hospitable to parasites. Additionally, adding a small amount of apple cider vinegar to your pet's water can help make their skin less appealing to fleas and ticks.

Natural Repellents Natural repellents like garlic and brewer's yeast can be added to your pet's diet. These substances can make your pet less appealing to fleas and ticks when consumed regularly. However, be sure to use these in moderation and consult with a veterinarian to avoid any adverse effects.

Home Remedies Home remedies like lemon sprays can also be effective. Boil sliced lemons in water, let the solution steep overnight, and spray it on your pet's fur. The citrus oils in lemons can repel fleas and other pests.

Using natural treatments for external parasites not only protects your pets and family from the potential side effects of chemical treatments but also supports a healthier, more eco-friendly approach to pest control. By incorporating these herbal sprays, essential oils, and preventative measures, you can effectively manage and prevent external parasite infestations naturally.

LONG-TERM PREVENTION

Ensuring long-term prevention of external parasites requires a multi-faceted approach. By maintaining a clean living environment, conducting regular inspections, and utilizing natural preventative measures, you can significantly reduce the risk of infestations and keep your home and pets healthy and parasite-free.

Maintaining a Clean Living Environment

Keeping your living space clean is paramount in preventing external parasites like fleas, ticks, lice, and mites. These pests thrive in dirty, cluttered environments, making regular cleaning and proper sanitation critical.

Regular Cleaning Regular vacuuming is essential, particularly in areas where pets sleep or spend most of their time. Vacuuming helps remove fleas, eggs, and larvae from carpets, upholstery, and cracks in floors. After vacuuming, dispose of the vacuum bag or empty the canister outside your home to prevent reinfestation.

Washing Bedding and Fabrics Frequently wash pet bedding, blankets, and any fabric items your pets use. Use hot water and a high-temperature dryer setting to kill any parasites and their eggs. Consider adding a few drops of essential oils like lavender or eucalyptus to the wash cycle for added repellency.

Yard Maintenance Maintain your yard by regularly mowing the lawn, trimming bushes, and removing debris where parasites might hide. This is especially important for preventing ticks and fleas. You can also use natural yard sprays containing cedar oil, which is effective in repelling many types of pests.

Regular Inspection and Early Detection

Early detection of external parasites can prevent an infestation from becoming severe. Regular inspections help catch problems before they escalate.

Pet Inspections Regularly inspect your pets for signs of parasites. Part the fur and check areas like the neck, behind the ears, and between the toes. Look for fleas, ticks, lice, and mite infestations. If you notice any unusual scratching, hair loss, or visible parasites, take action immediately.

Home Inspections Perform routine checks of your home, particularly in areas where pets frequent. Look for signs of pests, such as flea dirt, which looks like black pepper flakes, or tick nests in corners and under furniture. Use sticky traps to monitor for fleas and other insects.

Professional Pest Control Consider periodic inspections by a professional pest control service. They can provide a thorough assessment and recommend treatments if necessary. Many pest control services now offer natural and pet-safe options.

Natural Preventative Measures

Utilizing natural preventative measures can help keep external parasites at bay without the use of harsh chemicals. These methods are safer for your pets, family, and the environment.

Diatomaceous Earth Diatomaceous earth (DE) is a natural powder made from fossilized algae. It's non-toxic and safe for pets and humans when used correctly. Sprinkle DE on carpets, pet bedding, and outdoor areas. It works by dehydrating and killing parasites. Ensure you use food-grade DE and apply it lightly to avoid respiratory irritation.

Essential Oils Essential oils like lavender, eucalyptus, and cedarwood have natural insect-repelling properties. Create a spray by diluting these oils in water and use it around your home and on pet bedding. Be cautious when using essential oils on pets; always dilute them and consult a veterinarian for guidance.

Herbal Collars and Sachets Herbal collars and sachets can be an effective way to keep parasites away from your pets and home. These can be made with herbs like rosemary, thyme, and peppermint, which repel fleas and ticks. Place sachets in areas where pets sleep or use herbal collars for a constant deterrent.

Brewer's Yeast and Garlic Adding brewer's yeast and a small amount of garlic to your pet's diet can help make their blood less appealing to fleas and ticks. However, be sure to consult with a veterinarian before introducing garlic, as it can be harmful in large quantities.

Regular Grooming Regular grooming not only keeps your pets clean but also helps detect and remove parasites before they establish themselves. Use a flea comb to check for and remove fleas and ticks. Bathing your pets with natural shampoos containing neem oil or tea tree oil can also help repel pests.

By maintaining a clean living environment, conducting regular inspections, and using natural preventative measures, you can effectively manage and prevent external parasite infestations. These steps will help ensure a healthier, more comfortable living space for both you and your pets.

Conclusion

Managing external parasites demands a holistic approach that blends awareness, prevention, and natural treatments. By understanding these pests and their health impacts, you can proactively protect yourself and your loved ones. Regular inspections, early detection, and maintaining a clean environment are crucial for preventing infestations. Natural treatments such as herbal sprays and essential oils offer safe, effective alternatives to chemical solutions. Long-term prevention requires ongoing commitment to routine practices and staying informed about best strategies. By remaining vigilant, knowledgeable, and proactive, you can effectively manage external parasites and create a healthier, more comfortable living space for everyone in your household.

11. Psycho-Emotional Support During Parasite Cleanse

Engaging in a parasite cleanse can be a demanding and, at times, overwhelming experience. The physical effects of the cleanse, combined with the emotional and psychological stressors, necessitate comprehensive psycho-emotional support. Understanding how to manage stress and anxiety, incorporating mindfulness and meditation techniques, and seeking emotional support can significantly enhance the cleansing process and overall well-being.

MANAGING STRESS AND ANXIETY

The process of eliminating parasites from the body can be stressful. The physical symptoms and die-off reactions can trigger anxiety and exacerbate stress levels. To manage this, it's essential to recognize the sources of stress and implement strategies to mitigate them.

One effective approach is to maintain a routine. Establishing a daily schedule that includes time for relaxation, exercise, and adequate sleep can help regulate stress levels. Exercise, in particular, is beneficial as it releases endorphins, which are natural stress relievers. Engaging in moderate physical activities like walking, yoga, or swimming can provide significant relief from anxiety.

Another crucial aspect is to maintain a balanced diet. Certain foods, like those rich in magnesium (such as leafy greens, nuts, and seeds), can help reduce anxiety levels. Avoiding caffeine and sugar, which can exacerbate stress, is also advisable. Staying hydrated and consuming herbal teas, such as chamomile or lavender, can promote relaxation.

MINDFULNESS AND MEDITATION TECHNIQUES

Mindfulness and meditation can be valuable during a parasite cleanse. These practices help reduce stress and increase emotional resilience by focusing on the present moment. Simple techniques like mindful breathing can calm the mind and ease anxiety, and can be done anywhere.

Meditation is another powerful tool. Setting aside just 10-15 minutes each day for meditation can create a profound sense of peace and relaxation. Guided meditations, available through various apps and online platforms, can be particularly helpful for beginners. Techniques like progressive muscle relaxation, where you tense and then relax different muscle groups, can also relieve physical tension and promote mental calmness.

EMOTIONAL SUPPORT DURING THE CLEANSING PROCESS

Emotional support is vital when undergoing a parasite cleanse. Sharing your experiences with others who understand what you're going through can provide immense relief. Joining support groups, whether in-person or online, allows you to connect with others facing similar challenges. These groups offer a platform to share tips, encouragement, and empathy.

Communicating with family and friends about your cleanse journey is also important. Letting them know what you're experiencing can foster understanding and support. Sometimes, just having someone to listen can make a significant difference.

Professional help from a therapist can be crucial. They can offer coping strategies for stress and anxiety. Techniques like cognitive-behavioral therapy can help manage negative thoughts and maintain positivity during the cleanse process.

INCORPORATING SELF-CARE PRACTICES

Self-care is crucial during a parasite cleanse. Simple practices like taking a warm bath with Epsom salts, using essential oils like lavender or eucalyptus, and engaging in hobbies that bring joy can significantly improve your emotional well-being. Ensuring you get enough rest and sleep is also paramount, as your body needs time to heal and rejuvenate.

Engaging in creative activities, such as journaling, painting, or playing a musical instrument, can provide an emotional outlet and reduce stress. These activities allow you to express your feelings and thoughts in a constructive manner.

Conclusion

A parasite cleanse affects both body and mind. Managing stress, practicing mindfulness, and seeking support are key. These strategies can improve your overall well-being and help you navigate the cleanse more effectively. Remember, mental and emotional health are as crucial as physical aspects during this process.

12. Conclusion

REFLECTIONS ON THE IMPORTANCE OF NATURAL PARASITE CLEANSE

In reflecting on the journey through the world of natural parasite cleansing, it's evident that the importance of these practices extends far beyond merely addressing physical symptoms. The process of cleansing parasites naturally speaks to a broader philosophy of health and wellness that values the body's innate ability to heal and maintain balance when supported by natural, holistic methods.

Parasites, often unseen and undiagnosed, can have profound impacts on overall health. They can drain energy, disrupt digestion, and even affect mental well-being. Addressing these issues through natural methods is not only about eradicating the parasites but also about nurturing the body's systems to restore and maintain optimal health. Herbs, supplements, and dietary adjustments are more than just treatments; they are tools that empower individuals to take control of their health in a sustainable and non-invasive manner.

The significance of natural parasite cleanses also lies in their preventive potential. Regular cleanses and the integration of anti-parasitic foods and herbs into daily routines help create an internal environment that is inhospitable to parasites. This proactive approach reduces the risk of infections and promotes long-term wellness, highlighting the principle that prevention is always better than cure.

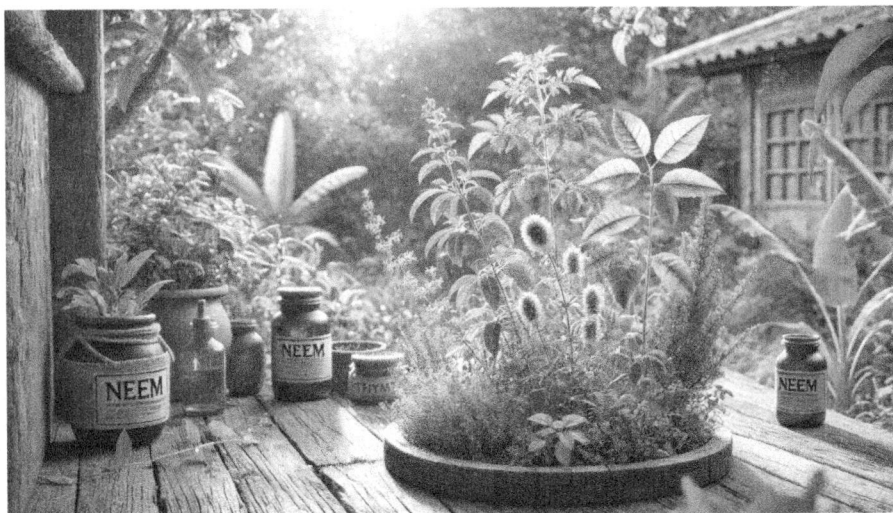

Moreover, the practices of natural parasite cleansing reconnect us with traditional knowledge and remedies that have been used for centuries across various cultures. This connection to ancient wisdom enriches our understanding of health, emphasizing the importance of respecting and preserving these time-tested practices.

The journey towards a parasite-free body is also an emotional and psychological endeavor. The process often involves overcoming fears and anxieties, dealing with uncomfortable symptoms, and maintaining commitment to the regimen. The psycho-emotional support, mindfulness, and stress reduction techniques discussed in this book are integral to a successful cleanse, underscoring the holistic nature of true healing.

CALL TO ACTION AND CONTINUED AWARENESS

As we conclude, remember that natural parasite cleansing is the beginning of a lifelong health journey. Use this knowledge for current concerns and future prevention. Start with small changes in diet and cleansing routines. Stay informed about natural health developments. Share your experiences to educate others and contribute to holistic health awareness. Regularly monitor your body and use learned diagnostic techniques.

Embrace a proactive, natural health-focused lifestyle. This approach not only protects your health but also promotes a shift towards sustainable wellness practices. Your commitment to natural cleansing reflects the power of nature and human resilience. Continue nurturing this commitment, stay informed, and inspire wellness in your community, fostering a healthier future where natural practices are part of everyday life.

Acknowledgments

This book would not have been possible without the support, knowledge, and encouragement of many individuals. First and foremost, I extend my deepest gratitude to my family for their unwavering support and belief in the importance of holistic health. Their patience and understanding have been invaluable throughout this journey.

Special thanks to the herbalists, naturopaths, and wellness experts who have generously shared their knowledge and expertise. Your insights have enriched this book and made it a more comprehensive resource for readers.

I am also grateful to the countless individuals who have shared their personal experiences with natural parasite cleansing. Your stories of healing and resilience are a source of inspiration and hope for others embarking on this path.

To my readers, thank you for your trust and commitment to natural health practices. May this book serve as a guide and companion on your journey to wellness. Your dedication to learning and applying these principles is a testament to the power of nature and the resilience of the human spirit.

Finally, I acknowledge the traditional healers and ancient wisdom that have laid the foundation for the practices discussed in this book. Your knowledge has transcended generations and continues to guide us in our pursuit of health and balance.

This book is a labor of love, born from a desire to empower individuals to take control of their health naturally. I hope it provides you with the knowledge, tools, and confidence to lead a healthier, parasite-free life.

Liv Marwin

Appendix

GLOSSARY OF TERMS

To ensure a comprehensive understanding of the topics discussed in this book, this glossary provides definitions for key terms related to natural parasite cleansing and holistic health practices. Familiarize yourself with these terms to enhance your grasp of the concepts presented.

Adaptogen: A natural substance considered to help the body adapt to stress and exert a normalizing effect upon bodily processes.

Anthelmintic: A type of drug or natural remedy used to expel or destroy parasitic worms.

Anti-parasitic: Referring to substances or treatments that kill or inhibit the growth of parasites.

Detoxification: The process of removing toxic substances or qualities.

Die-off Reaction: Also known as a Herxheimer reaction, it occurs when large quantities of toxins are released into the body as bacteria (or parasites) die during antibiotic treatment, causing a range of symptoms.

Ectoparasites: Parasites that live on the external surface of the host, such as fleas, ticks, lice, and mites.

Endoparasites: Parasites that live inside the host's body, such as intestinal worms and protozoa.

Herbal Infusion: A method of extracting the medicinal qualities of herbs by steeping them in hot water, oil, or alcohol.

Holistic Health: An approach to wellness that considers the whole person—body, mind, spirit, and emotions.

Immune-Boosting: Referring to actions, supplements, or foods that support or enhance the functioning of the immune system.

Probiotics: Live bacteria and yeasts that are beneficial for digestive health.

Protozoa: Single-celled microscopic organisms that can cause diseases, such as Giardia or Plasmodium (malaria).

Symbiosis: Interaction between two different organisms living in close physical association, typically to the advantage of both.

Tincture: An alcohol-based extract of a plant or herb.

Toxin: A poisonous substance produced within living cells or organisms.

ANTI-PARASITIC NUTRITIONAL GUIDE

Food Item	Nutrients	Anti-Parasitic Properties
Garlic	Allicin Sulfur	Effective against a range of parasites; boosts immunity
Pumpkin Seeds	Zinc Magnesium	Paralyzes parasites, aiding in their removal
Papaya Seeds	Enzymes Fiber	Contains proteolytic enzymes that kill parasites
Turmeric	Curcumin	Anti-inflammatory and anti-parasitic properties
Coconut Oil	Lauric Acid	Antimicrobial and antifungal properties
Cloves	Eugenol	Kills parasite eggs and larvae
Ginger	Gingerol	Improves digestion, fights parasites
Thyme	Thymol	Antiseptic, helps eliminate parasites
Cayenne Pepper	Capsaicin	Increases metabolism, expels parasites

These foods not only contribute to the elimination of parasites but also support overall health and wellness. Incorporating them into your daily diet can help maintain a balanced internal environment less conducive to parasitic infestations.

Thank You for Investing in Your Health!

We're thrilled you've chosen
"The Ultimate Guide to Parasite Cleanse."

CLAIM YOUR FREE GIFT

Discover nature's most powerful allies against parasites!
Scan to Get Your Free E-book

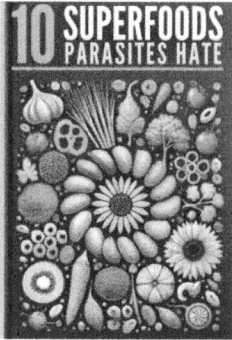

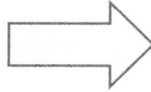

Share Your Success
Has this book improved your life?
Help others by sharing your experience.
Your review could be the nudge someone needs to start their own
health journey.

SCAN TO LEAVE A REVIEW

Remember, your health journey doesn't end here. Keep exploring, keep
learning, and keep thriving!

P.S. Join our community of health enthusiasts! Follow us on social media
for daily tips, success stories, and exclusive content to support your
ongoing wellness journey.

Facebook @MarwinBooks

Made in the USA
Las Vegas, NV
07 May 2025